"There is No Health Without Mental Health Anthology"

Men and Mental Health

Volume 2 - Series 3

True empowering, encouraging, and courageous lived experiences shared to inspire the world to "Stop the Stigma" around Mental Health and highlight There is no Health, without Mental Health.

Thank you all for sharing your journey and story!

Our people defeated Satan because of the blood of the Lamb and the message of God. They were willing to give up their lives. Revelations 12:11

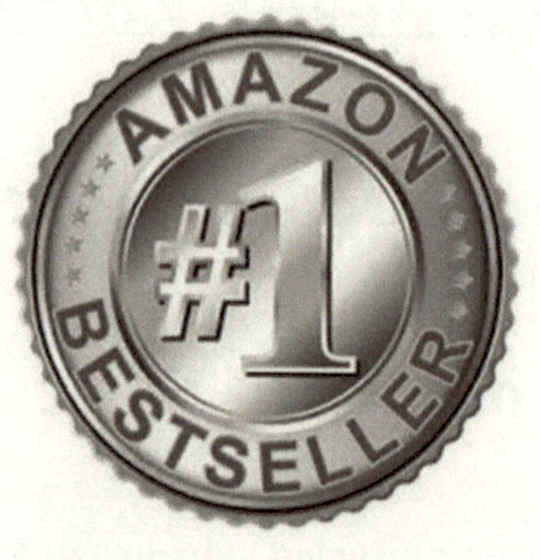

AMAZON
#1
BESTSELLER

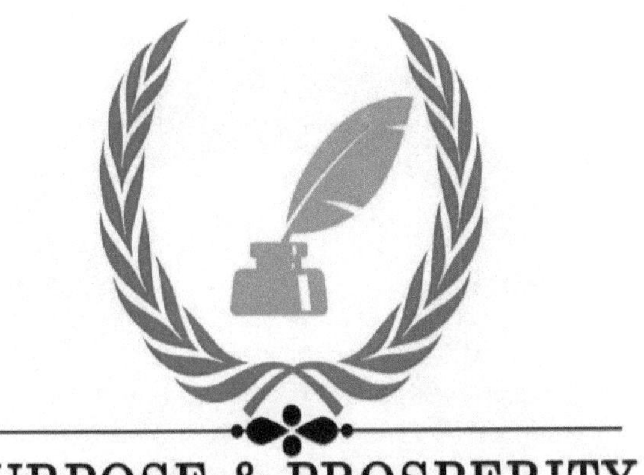

PURPOSE & PROSPERITY

PUBLISHING COMPANY ™

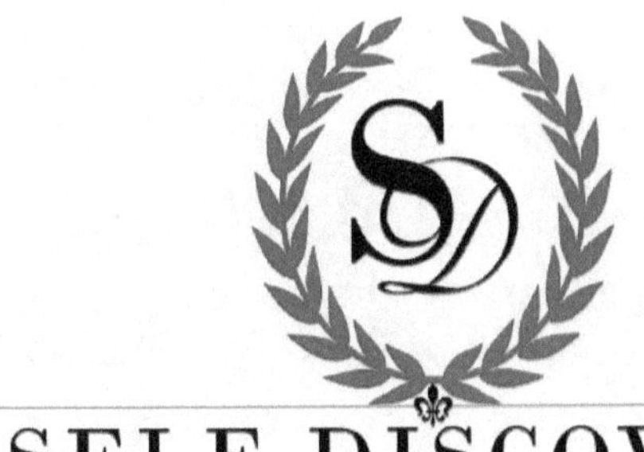

SELF-DISCOVERY

PAIN, POSITIONING AND PURPOSE, INC ™

**MENTAL HEALTH, SUICIDE PREVENTION
& CRISIS INTERVENTION SERVICES.**

NATIONAL
SUICIDE
PREVENTION
LIFELINE
1-800-273-TALK (8255)
suicidepreventionlifeline.org

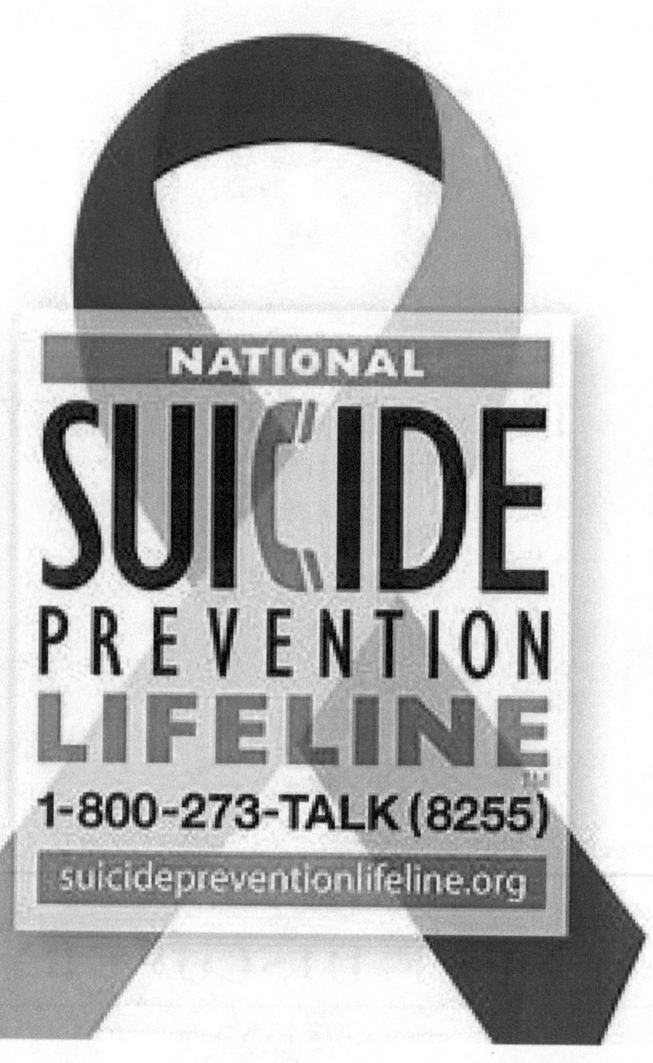

Dial 988

Dedication

This book is dedicated to my older brother, a Decorated Army Veteran, the Veterans, Soldiers, and those perished by way of suicide. Their life and legacy will live on through those of us that boldly and courageously fight the stigma that is attached to mental illness.

You matter. All lives matter.

No Silence. No Stigma. No Suicide.

We are, The Voices Behind Mental Illness.

Authors, let us BOLDLY SPEAK

on the importance of Mental Health and Wellness

&

Suicide Prevention.

Each One, Reach One. Reach One, Teach One.

Table of Contents

Table of Contents – Con't.

Introduction

One area that often goes ignored by men is mental health. In fact, suicide has become a silent killer for men, with statistics showing us that men are nearly four times more likely to die by suicide than women. This trend is proof that men need to start taking their mental health seriously.

According to the American Foundation for Suicide Prevention, men are 3.54 times more likely to die by suicide than women. Men, in fact, account for almost 70% of all suicides.

There are a multitude of stresses facing men that contribute to or exacerbate mental health illness. Financial pressures, supporting a family, and juggling a career are just a few of the day-to-day challenges that can affect a man's mood. The additional stressor of keeping a façade of strength, and not talking about these issues, only makes the problem worse.

Statistically, about 90% of people who dies by suicide have a diagnosable mental illness at the time of their death, most often depression. At the heart of depression in men lies a disinterest in the activities that used to bring you joy. Bad moods, apathy, an inability to sleep or sleeping too much are other signs of depression.

And in terms of anxiety, a feeling of persistent anxiousness, restlessness, or racing thoughts can all be present. A major challenge for men, can be differentiating between clinical depression and merely passing it off as a "bad mood".

While women are in fact diagnosed with depression at a much higher rate than men, the willingness to talk about their feelings may be very different, thus causing the symptoms to manifest differently. Men are less likely to speak up about their mental health struggles, often internalizing their pain. As men, we have been socialized to shy away from showing signs of weakness. We have been taught to "fight through" mental health issues. From early childhood we are told to "suck it up", and that "big boys don't cry". We have been socialized not to talk about our feelings. This attitude makes men more likely to discount serious symptoms. In the worst cases, they can go on to self-medicate with drugs and alcohol.

It is time to normalize men speaking up about their mental health, and to create safe spaces where men can voice their feelings without judgement. These spaces break down the stigma surrounding men and their feelings — and mean fewer men must suffer in silence. Talking about mental health puts men in a vulnerable position, which is understandably uncomfortable and often feels unnatural to a man who has been told all his life that sharing feelings indicates weakness, which is unbecoming. The key is teaching men to identify, understand, and respond to signs of mental illness, and to recognize that there is no weakness in acknowledging a need for help. To do this, men need safe spaces; low-pressure environments where they can open up to people they know and trust. In a best-case scenario, the safe space starts at home with loved ones, spouses, and partners, asking the men in their lives how they are feeling and recommending seeking help if there appears to be a persistent issue. Show that you're there, you're present, you're non-judgmental, and you're willing to help them through whatever they might be going through.

Acknowledging that you need help and asking for that help, opens a world of options, including therapy, medication, or some combination of both. And coping mechanisms such as changes to diet, exercise, or meditation are also viable options.

The statistics surrounding men's mental health can no longer be ignored. Changing the way men engage with their emotions is a crucial first step in terms of turning around these numbers. Opening up about our feelings and seeking out effective care is essential if we, as men, are going to live our lives to the fullest. As men, we owe it not only to those we love, but also to ourselves, to be the best version of ourselves that we can be. There is no value or valor in suffering alone, in silence. As men, it is time for us to be vocal, be vulnerable, and be visible as we create space for healing.

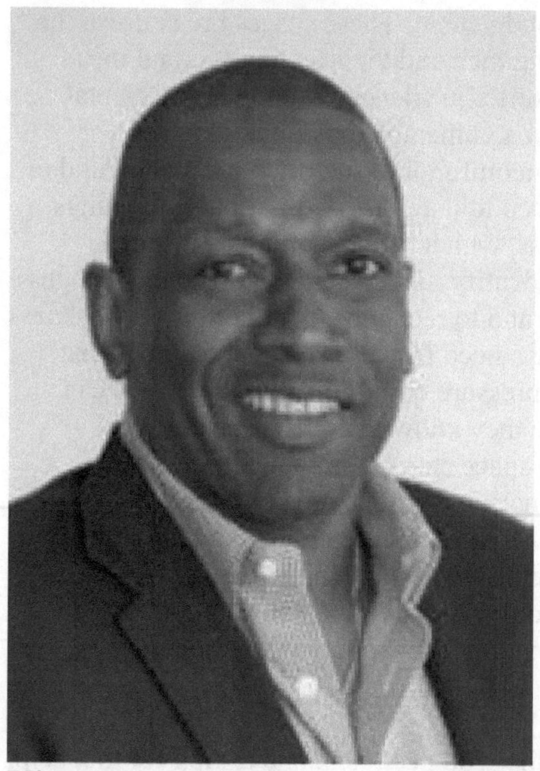

Victor Armstrong
Director of the NC Division of Mental Health,
Developmental Disabilities, and Substance Abuse Services

Biography

Victor Armstrong is Director of the NC Division of Mental Health, Developmental Disabilities, and Substance Abuse Services. Prior to this role, Victor spent six years as Vice President of Behavioral Health with Atrium Health where he had responsibility for operations of Atrium's largest behavioral health hospital, Behavioral Health Charlotte. Victor has over 30 years of experience in human services, primarily dedicated to building and strengthening community resources to serve individuals living with mental illness.

Victor currently serves on the board of directors of American Foundation for Suicide Prevention (AFSP) NC. He is also former board chair of NAMI NC, and a member of American Association of Suicidology (AAS), and NASW-NC. Victor is a former member of the Board of Directors of National Council for Behavioral Health, i2i Center for Integrative Health, and RI International.

Victor's awards and recognitions include 2019 Black Mental Health Symposium -Mental Health Advocate of the Year, 2019 Atrium Health Excellence in Diversity & Inclusion Award, 2018 Distinguished Alumni Award from East Carolina University School of Social Work, Pride Magazine 2018 "Best of the Best", and i2i Center for Integrative Health 2018 Innovation Award for "Whole Person Care", 2012 National Alliance on Mental Illness (NAMI) NC, Mental Health Professional of the Year.

Victor graduated, Magna Cum Laude, from North Carolina Central; University with a bachelor's degree in Business Management and received a Master of Social Work (MSW) from East Carolina University. He is the husband of Dr. Charletta Armstrong and the father of 3 sons, Carter, Alonzo, and Victor Jr.

Venessa's Prologue

The past ten years of my life has been a whirlwind, in which I must confess, it has been bittersweet, to say the least. My mother went to be with the Lord, September 1, 2000, her birthday is on September 30th and…. September 2016 my older brother, passed by way of suicide. This is when my mental health began to scream loudly internally, but silently externally. I too, was paralyzed by the stigma connected to mental illness. I thought, what would people think? Not to mention my family, how will they portray me? It was during this time I was introduced to physiotherapy, group therapy, in-patient and intensive outpatient treatment, as well as medication that continues to help me on my recovery journey. The stigma is what keeps people from admitting they need help and are struggling. Whilst we **all** have mental health, *why is it so hard to admit the struggle mentally, emotionally, and spiritually? Is it the same reason I gave above? Could it be you just didn't know? Or maybe you simply felt hopeless and thought there wasn't help and resources available?* I have great news for you. **YOU ARE NOT ALONE!** *For everyone has sinned; we all fall short of God's glorious standard. Romans 3:23* With support, hope, tools, and resources, you can make it. *With Christ, you can do all things but fail.* It is my *HOPE and PRAYER* that YOU will gain *COURAGE, STRENGTH, UNDERSTANDING, REVELATION* as well as *RESILIENCY* as you encounter the testimonies of men that speak their truth in transparency, without shame and stigma. Tighten your seat belt….This will be a RIDE!!

Let's Talk!!

Venessa D. Abram

FOREWORD

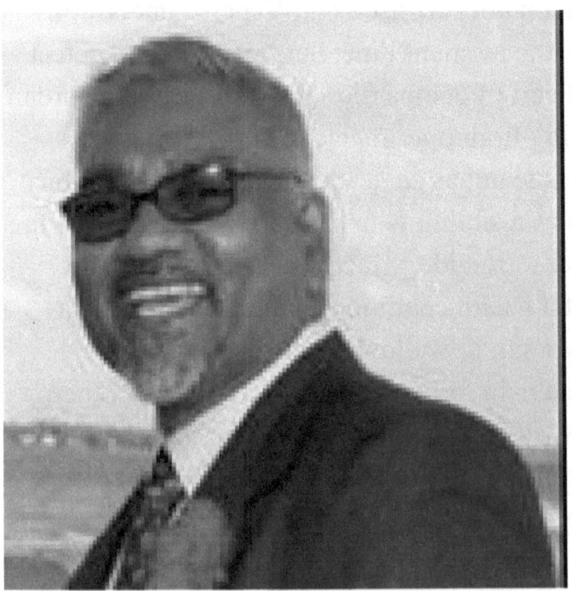

Dr. Donovan Thomas

It is indeed my delight to have been invited to write the Foreword for this important book, Men and Mental Health - Volume 2 – Series 3. My service to humanity over the last thirty plus years has exposed me to the demise and destruction of too many men, from all walks of life and all ages, who suffered from mental health conditions. My work and research in the field of suicide prevention has led to awareness that almost 90 percent of the almost 600,000 men who die by suicide annually have suffered from diagnosable mental health conditions. Almost 70 million people, consisting of family members, close friends, and associates, are left to grieve every year because of the death by suicide of a man in their lives with diagnosable mental health condition!

I wish to commend Venessa Abram, for having undertaken the important task of authoring this well-needed literary masterpiece. I am not surprised that Venessa undertook this task. From the moment I met her, I was able to detect that she has a heart of compassion for, and carried a burden for men suffering from poor mental health. Venessa, comes to this issue not as an academician nor as a curious researcher, but as a sibling who has suffered the pain of the loss of a brother to suicide, which was triggered by untreated mental health condition. Venessa has made a deliberate choice not to wallow in self-pity and be paralyzed by the pain following the death of her brother. Instead she has, against all odds, chosen to find purpose in the pain, which has been processed and continues to be processed, to provide a platform for purpose, fulfillment, and the healing of many lives.

Commendations are also in order to the brave purpose-driven men, who have unreservedly contributed their stories to this book. Your truth narratives of personal transformation add value and legitimacy to this work. Your literary pieces are inspirational, and I am convinced that as they are read, conviction and desire for change for the better will come to many broken lives. Thanks for this courageous contribution to the mental health and wellbeing of men! The input of Angela Washington, with the pertinent poetry adds a positive flavor to the flow and the text overall. Our author, Venessa Abram, has chosen wisely in having invited Dr. Victor Armstrong to contribute the introduction. I echo Dr. Armstrong's call that the time has come, *'to normalize men speaking up about their mental health… without judgment."*

As I survey various chapters in the book, I am once again enthralled by the power of God to change lives. As you read Brian Anderson's journey you won't miss the miraculous work of God to protect this 13th man. Read Kamua Sullivan's story and *learn about that which gave him peace of mind and confidence in the midst of a troubled life. Spend the time to travel the road of recovering with Sullivan and celebrate that even the man who struggles with mental health issues can be empowered to help the broken, battered and bruised. The reflections of Dempris Gasque will encourage honesty and hope as we traverse this life. I encourage you to read the entire book and may you find the courage and strength to see possibilities and experience breakthrough, even in the midst of the unpleasant realities of mental health.*

Mental health issues have been impacting men from time immemorial. This book has much relevance as this issue of mental health of men continues to be a challenge in our world today. Yet this issue is often shrouded in secrecy and even denial. There are several prevailing factors that do not encourage men to give attention to their mental wellbeing. Chief among these is the stigma associated with this illness. Yes, I did say illness … and many times it is treated as a curse and not as an illness. Often times the man refuses to disclose his need for help because of his fear of rejection. On other occasions psychological factors prevent him from coming to the fore to seek help. He would rather internalize than discloses his need for mental health assistance. Whatever the reasons for the silence and secrecy regarding men and mental health, Venessa Abram and her contributing authors, have now exposed this important issue that has been buried for too long.

Let's face the reality. *We are losing too many of our men because of unattended mental health issues. It is time for us to rise up, reject the unhealthy practices and renew our passion to play our part in eradicating the silence surrounding men and mental health. You have an important part to play.*

Again, I applaud Venessa Abram for the service she has done in producing this significant well-timed work.

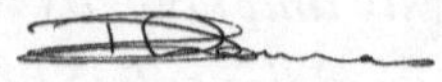

Dr. Donovan Thomas
President,
Choose Life International

Chapter I.

Silence is not a Cure

Being strong,
is what I do.
Being strong,
is nothing new.
Smiling through,
the good and bad.
Standing firm,
when times are sad.
Holding back,
the pain I feel.
Hiding thoughts,
that seem unreal.
Seeing things,
that are not there.
I know inside,
no one will care.
Schizo stupid!
That's what they'll say.
I'll just be quiet,
sit down and pray.

Angela
Washington

Chapter II.

#13

Brian Anderson

Mark 11:1-3: Describes the scene, when Jesus was planning his triumphant journey into Jerusalem; he told two of the disciples to go to this particular farmhouse to get this particular donkey. Then Jesus says: Now the donkey that I want you to get   Make sure it's the one that has been tied up all his life…. Make sure it's the one that has never been ridden… that means it was untamed! Then Jesus said this amazing thing, if the people there ask you why I chose that donkey, tell them "I HAVE NEED OF HIM". I relate to that donkey in so many ways; tied up; never ridden; untamed; wild. Jesus told Satan years ago, "leave Brian Keith Anderson alone". "I HAVE NEED OF HIM".

I have need of Him.

I want to share with you a story, a true-life narrative of 13 different men. A story based around the # 13. 13 different people, from 13 different Christian families. All 13 went to Christian church schools, all 13 had great futures ahead of them, All 13 had one thing in common, that thing was, all 13 suffered from mental illness and or addictive disease. Let's see what happened to these 13. Two were executed via the electric chair (still in the struggle), Two were killed by gunshot (still in the struggle), One died in a deadly car crash (still in the struggle), One died by suicide (still in the struggle), One died from an overdose (still in the struggle), One died on drugs (still in the struggle), One died from AIDS (still in the struggle), One is currently dying today from AIDS (still in the struggle), Two are yet (still in the struggle.) So, the statistics are clear, 69.23 % of those Christian raised men died before they were ever rescued.

Wait a minute, that only adds up to 12 men, what happened to the # 13?

13 found himself homeless at the age of five with his father and two older brothers. # 13 was molested at the age of seven and eight years old. # 13 found himself homeless over and over again from the age of eight to eleven or twelve years old with his father and two older brothers. # 13 remembers one of the worst times being homeless was living in Huntsville Ala. Once again # 13 was homeless with his father and two older brothers. The father found an abandon trailer on the side of the road, with cardboard taped to the broken windows. It was the dead of winter, no heat, no electricity, no running water, and to make matters worse, there was a huge hole in the floor where the cold air came flowing through. The only thing in the trailer was a box spring and mattress. # 13s father would lay them all down on the box spring and pull the mattress on top of them all; so, they wouldn't freeze to death at night. # 13 was teased and ridiculed for being the stinky, dirty, and dumb kid in school. # 13 developed an undiagnosed mental illness from all the trauma he experienced as a child. # 13 turned to drugs at the age of seventeen. # 13 became addicted at the age of eighteen and at the same time found himself homeless again. # 13 had his first suicide attempt at the age of nineteen.

13 would end up in jail on three different occasions from the age of twenty to twenty- four. # 13 became a stone-cold drug addict by then. # 13 had his second suicide attempt at the age of twenty- six. # 13 was facing long term jail or lockdown inpatient treatment at that same age. # 13 ended up in lockdown inpatient treatment for 28 days. # 13 found his God, himself and recovery while locked away in

treatment. # 13 got out of treatment FIRED UP about recovery. # 13 would tell his story everywhere he went. # 13 started being recognized for his passion and his story. # 13 was asked to speak all over the country from Seattle Washington to Palo Alto California, from Utah to Texas, from Orlando to Baltimore etc. etc. # 13 was asked to speak on TBN twice, Atlanta Live twice, local TV and Radio station in the Augusta Ga. Area. # 13 wrote two books on Hope and Recovery "Beautiful Scars, My Journey to Wholeness and Healing" and "Beautiful Scars Two, The Ripple Effect." # 13 Books have made their way to South Africa, Japan, the UK etc. # 13s books have been endorsed by leading Meatal Health and Addiction Professionals etc.

13 founded his own 501c3 "Beautiful Scars Inc." where our motto is "Come to us with open wounds, Leave with BEAUTIFUL SCARS."

So. what happened to # 13?

13 just finished writing this article. Hello, my name is Brian Keith Anderson AKA # 13, and I HAVE A STORY TO TELL. The beauty of my story and the tens of thousands like me is that we get a chance to give back to the thing that almost killed us all. It's one thing to read about hope and recovery in a book, or hear about it in an article, movie, or TV show, it's another thing to be in the presence of one who has lived it. There's a connection that takes place like none other. I speak from experience. Curtis Graham was the first person that showed me recovery is possible by sharing his recovery journey with me. It literally changed my life.

For the first time I saw hope and recovery standing right in front of me… Then and only then would I KNOW that it is possible. Notice I said "KNOW" it is possible, I didn't say I believed it was possible. There's a difference in "believing" and "KNOWING." All beliefs can be debated, but what you KNOW you KNOW. One of the definitions of the word "KNOW" is (To have an intimate relationship with.) Once Curtis Graham 1. Told me, then he 2. Showed me, and then 3. I tried it and it worked.

I've had the privilege of receiving several Certifications in the field of Mental Health. I'm very proud of all my accomplishments and the hard work it took to gain them. But what I'm most proud of is the title I've given myself "Mountain Climber." You see I've had to climb some mighty mountains in my life time such as Homelessness, Molestation, Mental Illness, Drug Addiction, 3-time jail, 2 Suicide Attempts, Lockdown Inpatient Treatment for 28 days and so on and so on… I will end with the parable of "The Mountain Climber."

There was a Preacher, a Doctor and a Mountain Climber that showed up at the gates of Heaven. Gabriel was standing at the gate with a bag filled with wings. The Preacher walks before Gabriel, Gabriel reaches into the bag, Gabriel pulls out 2 wings. Gabriel pins the 2 wings on the back of the Preacher, then Gabriel says "Now perform for me, and prove to me that you're worthy to enter the gate." That Preacher started flapping both his wings, took off into the air, did a beautiful spin, came down and landed, Gabriel said "Enter thou in, for you have proven yourself worthy to walk through the gate."

The Doctor walks before Gabriel, Gabriel reaches into the bag, Gabriel pulls out 2 wings, Gabriel pins those 2 wings on the back of the Doctor, Gabriel says "Now perform for me, and prove to me that you're worthy to walk through the gate." That Doctor starts flapping those 2 wings, that Doctor takes off into the air, that Doctor does a beautiful spin, that Doctor comes down and lands, Gabriel says

"Enter thou in, for you have proven yourself worthy to walk through the gate."

The Mountain Climber walks before Gabriel, Gabriel reaches into the bag, Gabriel pulls out 1 wing, Gabriel pins that 1 wing on the back of that Mountain Climber, then Gabriel says "Now perform for me, and prove to me that you're worthy to walk through the gate." Just then every Mountain that that Mountain Climber had to climb in his life time came rushing back to his memory. That Mountain Climber started flapping that 1 wing, that Mountain Climber taxies to the beginning of that runway, that Mountain Climber flapped that 1 wing some more, That Mountain Climber takes off down that runway, shoots up into the air, that Mountain Climber did a spin, a turn, a flip, some somersaults, some more spins, some more turns, some more flips, some more somersaults…. Just then an Angel walked up to Gabriel and said "Gabriel, who in the heavens is that.? Gabriel says "That's the Mountain Climber, showing what you can do with HALF THE CHANCE."

So, the next time someone walks up to me and says "Wasn't you diagnosed with a mental illness, in jail 3 times, 2 suicide attempts and a drug addict? What gives you the right to smile and think you have something to say? I shrug my shoulder back, look them dead in the eyes and say "ONE WING BABY, ONE WING."

Journey Booklist

Battlefield of the Mind- Joyce Meyers

The Lioness Arising- Lisa Bevere

The Alchemist- Paul Coelho

Confident Woman- Joyce Meyers

The Awakened Woman – Dr. Tererai Trent

The Art of War- Sun Tzu

The Magic of Thinking Big- David J. Schwarts, Ph.D.

Therapist:

https://therapyforblackgirls.com/

Biography

Brian Keith Anderson is the Administrator of Peer Support Services for Behavioral Health Link (BHL); a Certified Peer Specialist/Certified Recovery Educator (CPS/CRE), Certified Whole Health and Wellness Coach, Certified WRAP facilitator, Certified Mental Health First Aid Trainer and Co-Founder of Beautiful Scars, Inc. In addition to this, he is an author who has a genuine compassion for those in need.

Life hasn't always been easy. At the age of 5, he found himself homeless along with his father and two older brothers. Sleeping in a car with no money, no food and not knowing what was going to happen next. Periodically a family would allow them to sleep on their floor for a couple of days. However, as time passed, they found themselves homeless again. Around the age of 7 or 8, Brian was molested by a member of one of the families that took them off the streets. This secret was kept from his family and father because he didn't want them to be homeless, living in a car without warmth or food. Due to the molestation and chronic homelessness, his learning suffered, and he was ridiculed by the other students because he couldn't read or write well. In addition to this, he was known as the "smelly" little boy. Because of being homeless, there wasn't money to buy soap, brush his teeth or wash his clothes.

All these occurrences led Brian on a spiraling road to mental illness, drug addiction, self-hatred, three times jailed, chronic homelessness as a young adult, two suicide attempts, lock down in- patient treatment and more.

With the help of God, a praying father, and a man who had been through what he was going through, changed came. Now Brian can proudly say that he has been on TBN twice, Atlanta Live twice, and several local tv and radio stations in Augusta, Georgia. His books have been endorsed by leading mental health professionals and are being utilized as teaching tools.

 As a person who has recovered from homelessness, hopelessness, drug addiction, molestation, mental illness, jail, suicidal ideation, and more, he has a strong devotion to helping others on their road to recovery and healing.

Beautiful Scars *"My journey to Wholeness and Healing"*

Brian chronicles his own journey to recovery, and shares in (often painful) detail how he fought a seemingly un-winnable battle with his own personal demons. Substance abuse and mental illness plunged him into the depths of darkness and despair, leading him to attempt suicide twice. Now he shares his message of hope and healing so that others who are traveling the road he traveled can also experience wholeness and freedom from the chains and shackles of mental illness and addiction.

Beautiful Scars 'Two' *The Ripple Effect*

Brian has poignantly detailed the significance of how one person can create a ripple effect in the lives of many for years to come. His inspirational words will reach into the deepest recesses of your heart and soul and ignite a flame of hope where there was despair.

You can find both his books on Amazon.com. Please view some of his inspirational work on www.Beautiful-scars.org. Click on videos. Brian Anderson can be reached at (706)231-9588.

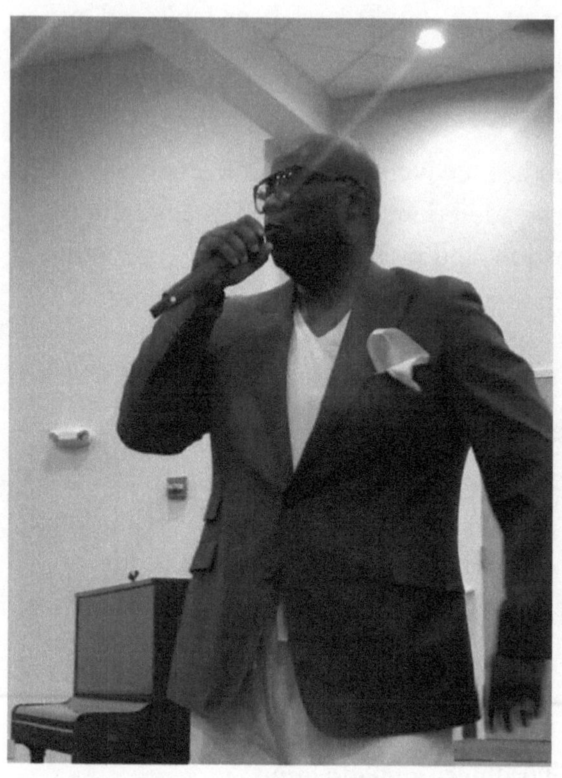

Chapter III.

Men and Their Mastery Over Themselves

Kamau Sullivan

"God is the vault within which I keep the treasure that is my humanity. I make withdrawals every day so that I can fulfill my obligation to respect, forgive, consider, and communicate with humanity. But I keep the best of me secure and uncontaminated with my Lord. In that sense, I cannot be robbed, cheated, or truly bankrupt. The best of me resides safely in a special account with my Creator. The interest accrued finances my hope, love, mercy, tolerance, and faith. In this sense... I am a wealthy man."

Kamau Sullivan

All humans share the common plight of investing in the building, investigating, monitoring, and repairing our... selves. However, there is something special that occurs in a young girl's life that exponentially propels her ahead of boys and even men with regards to maturity, self-awareness, and being in touch with reality. I am referring to the menstrual cycle. On that day, a young girl's transforms into a young woman whether she likes it or not. The reality of maturity, growing older, maintenance of the body, and the truth behind womanhood becomes real.

Meanwhile, boys remain immature, ignore everything about their bodies, and have no idea about the girl-to-young woman-to-woman journey. This, to me is the beginning of the great divide between men and women. Why does this matter? Because if we traveled the road to maturity, self-awareness, and the reality of our own biological evolutions, we would be less surprised by the respective needs, fears,

insecurities, and imperfections of our counterparts
(opposite sex). Instead we have this misconception,
unrealistic expectation, impatience, and sometimes
intolerance for the imperfection of each other. If the men
would mature enough to handle the truth, then the women
could retire from pretending to be the "perfect female" and
so the men could stop pretending to be the "perfect male."
Then perhaps we could all live with the truth about each
other.

It's the chicken and the egg, and no one can blame the
male or the female. However, any individual human can
make an effort to stop "playing the game." I mention this,
in order to propose the idea that we as humans play many
such games. Pretending is a game to the youth, but
pretending, with regards to critical matter, as an adult has
lead to dire circumstances concerning multiple aspects of
our lives (including mental health, sincere communication,
and a realistic perspective with regards to interacting with
self and others).

What is the male equivalent of the first menstrual event?
Oh, it's an event, alright - the very first time you wake up
in a pool of blood. So, what do boys have to wake them up
to the seriousness of reality with regards to their bodies,
emotions (and the concept of not always being in control of
their emotional state, and probability that males and
females are not some perfect barbie doll thing? Nothing.
Nothing like a first menstrual cycle. However, men have
women. We have moms, sisters, and we have the
researchable truth. The truth about women is not an
unsolvable mystery that cannot be effectively
communicated to men. Therefore, boys should not be left

behind, ignorant of this "heads up/warning" that reality is coming your way.

My premise is that boys are allowed to escape this monumental contact with reality and so they continue on with no need to mature at any particular rate. They are not exposed to their first stigma, nor are they aware that they mind and body are evolving in a way that is critical and that deserves attention, respect, maturity, and even medical care. By the time a man becomes aware that human bodies need medical checkups and self-examinations; they've already decided that women are crazy, high-maintenance, overly particular and so on. In that way, men have gotten used to stigmatizing women and believing themselves to be above such high-maintenance lifestyles. Until, that is, they are warned about their age, weight, prostate, colon, cholesterol, and blood pressure. By the time, a man is fifty years old... the damage is done. They view any interruption of their perfectly fine life (zero need for medication or medical care) as something temporary or ignorable. This denial at this point in ones life can be powerful and blinding.

"I'm not an old lady. I'm not taking a bunch of pills. I'm grown, I don't need anyone telling me how I feel." And that's if he makes it to fifty. Men's disconnection with the needs, risks, and eventual decline of their bodies, in my opinion, starts the day their sister has her first menstrual cycle. On that day, the boys should be prompted to move forward with the girls; and it's the job of both parents to make this happen. On that day and from then on, a girl's mental and emotional capacity is required to make a series of huge jumps forward. For the boy... nothing has nor will change for decades. This emotional gapping is profoundly consequential and the consequences affect every aspect of male and female interactions.

What if I told you that a seed planted in soil that had no nutrients in it wouldn't grow? What if I told you that a fish swimming in a toxic pond wouldn't live long? What if I told you that a spouse married to an immature spouse might get a divorce? You would begin to see the correlation between anything that has needs or has vulnerabilities and the consequences of being surrounded by something insufficient or even harmful.

So, in a sense, I've written about the event that begins the divide between the genders. I've also indicated how critical I feel that the correlation is between that lost opportunity to learn and grow is to the overall cost/damage done to the connection between men and women. In the end, what is also created and lost is the ability to apply or deny the perception of a stigma, respectively. When we lose that connection, that mutual understanding and sense of need and vulnerability that is human, the power to apply and the inability to escape a stigma is born. Otherwise we are connected and no man reaches the age of seventeen without being ashamed to make jokes of a girl's menses, because "My mother and my sister have a cycle. Healthy women have a menses; so, I'm not sure I get the joke?".

It is my opinion, that this initial disconnect between the genders, leads to the ability for men to have, harbor, and even cherish a gross superiority complex over the women. Instead of empathy, an informed perspective, and a humble acceptance of reality, this detachment allows the men to hand out the stigmas as they see fit. Womanhood is one huge stigma in and of itself, but men who show any "symptoms" of womanhood are also assigned stigmas. So, if your need is voiced; you're needy. If you watch your language, what you eat, and avoid looking at women who aren't your wife... you're a prude. Don't get me wrong, if you hold women accountable to unrealistic expectations, so too, will the women expect an unrealistic version of men. Therefore, the stigmas fly both ways.

Pride, arrogance, a feeling of superiority, and the notion that one is less vulnerable or needy than others can be the sources of self-imposed stigmas. Once a person has declared themselves above weakness, then ever need is seen as a contradiction to their control of weakness. Maintaining control of ones weaknesses can quickly become a person's obsession; their purpose in life.

"The judge says that I beat my wife because I let anger control me. That can't be true because I am strong, not weak."

"The doctor says that I need medication to keep my mind from turning on itself. If I let meds run my mind then I am a slave to the doctor and his treatments."

While there is some validity to having a cautious perspective with regards to interference in one's life choices, a rational mind can distinguish between admonishment and advice or help and interference. Part of my purpose, within this essay, is to propose and explore one of the avenues of divergence between the social, mental, ethical, spiritual, and psychological connectedness that both genders share as humans. In my opinion, to continue to point, blame, analyze and generate possible solutions from one side or the other suppresses the mutual accountability and capacity of each gender as members of humanity. I refuse to do this, and in all my lifetime, I have always approached every problem, disagreement, and mystery between myself and any female from the perspective that we are both humans and we should both expect great things from each other.

Instead, there are some men and women who feel boxed into some category or another. Some feel as though they are being unrealistic in their resistance to settling for a quality friend, relationship with their parents, or spouse. Some feel as though no one can communicate with them on the level and depth that they need. Millions of men and women who feel this way and so the suppression and self-suppression that comes between us and doing the right thing occurs for both genders. I mention this because we are all in this together. We make it hard for each other. Humans are the oppressors and caretakers of humans.

How can we reach through the barricades the we put up between ourselves and the help, forgiveness, and improvement that we need? How can we reach through the barriers that others have erected in order to help them? Pride, arrogance, a feeling of superiority, and the notion that one is less vulnerable or needy are just a few of the less subtle obstacles faced by those who wish to help themselves and others. Trust issues, communication issues, perception issues, and a desire to keep private matters private are a few of the more subtle obstacles. Other hindrances include a certainty that others won't understand, won't be sincere or consistent in their desire to help, or a hopelessness in the possibility to correct or improve a condition or situation (especially an addiction). It makes no sense to separate these issues, obstacles, or perspectives with regards to genders. It makes more sense to attack the source, perceived need/benefits, and counter logic that will help someone breakthrough in order to provide help (and the recipient to receive and utilize that help). Or is it the case that a solution for one gender only works for that gender? Then is it the case that what appears to be an issue, or condition is actually a gender-based issue or condition? Is the mental or physical abuse of a girl going to result in a different set of issues than it would when the same abuse happens to a boy? Do girls who have been mentally or physically abused develop distinctly different issues/conditions than do boys who develop into men (having suffered those same abuses)?

Allow me to clarify my purpose and thus intention behind the questions above. I'm not interested in the debate as to weather males and females suffer the same way and thus need the same methods of treatment or assistance. Literally, the opposite, I mean to focus on the source of the issues, initiation of the building of the obstacles that prevent effective treatment, as well as the vast avenues and options that we as humans can generate in order to help other humans. In a sense, I'm belittling all things not the problem and the solution in order to show a disdain for every excuse for not effectively administering and receiving the help that each of us needs. And as I mentioned from the beginning, we, as humans, all need help throughout our lifespans.

The differences between the genders are real and beautiful. But how men and women come to view each other and the other's issues as being so disparate, mysterious, and unconquerable is as much a shame as it is a sham. I mentioned that I believe the disparity and division originates with the powerful (to the girls and a nonoccurrence to boys) event that is a young girl's first menstruation. It's a natural and highly personal experience. It makes sense that the boys are left out of it, especially little, immature boys. The point is not to make the experience a family matter, the point is that the event marks a point in time in which parents can accept that their children aren't always going to be babies and the parenting needs to be leveled up for all the children in that family. Now is the time for setting standard for equality, reinforcing the benefit in seeking help and communicating truthfully. An entire family setting the best example as a family. Otherwise... we wait. We wait and the various diseases of the heart and mind go untreated, grow unchallenged, and become an unstoppable force that dominates the intellect and destroys every possible relationship.

The issues that affect humanity are vast. From geopolitical neglect and disdain between countries and apathy and violence between neighbors, to the insidious deterioration of love between spouses; we humans have some profoundly serious work to do.

To deny that humans are a multi-layered and evolving conglomeration of experiences, emotions, capacity, and perspectives is to deny the complex processes involved in untangling those aspects of the one who is in distress. The complex nature of human perception, interaction, reaction, and the processing/interpretation of the sum of their day-to-day experiences speaks to the aspect of individuality that is the common plight of all humans. We all experience. We all misinterpret some things, sometimes. We all suffer. We all cope with a list of burdens. We all press on, pushing our pain thresholds a bit higher. We all need a good friend. We all need to be understood. We all have a incredible story to tell.

Humans. Humanity... we forget that it is a common plight with a common solution. In our struggle to love our own uniqueness, to love our special selves, and to do so despite being unappreciated for who we are, categorized for how we are, and even despised for the way we are, we separate ourselves from the two components of the grand solution. Each other and God. We treat each other so poorly that we give up on humanity and we feel so alone that we end up distancing ourselves from our Creator. Indeed, we have been created to be complex creatures, but the wounds and the treatment for those wounds are quite simple. We have fooled ourselves into thinking that the source of our troubles are as complex as the times, the technologies, and our complicated make up.

Map to Mental Wellness Success

My recipe for sanity amidst the madness, sincerity in my hope for society, and a snuggly love for myself is as simple as I need it to be. Meaning, if I pretend it works then it fails. If it works, I don't pretend that it needs to be more complex. I never end a night or begin a morning without prayer. I surround myself with only good people. When I cannot find a good person, I patiently use my solitude to improve myself so that when I'm blessed to find a good person, I am good for them. Finally, I put my hope and trust with regards to my deepest needs, desires, and fears all in one place. A place where no one else can get to them (to use them against me). God is the vault within which I place all of my humanity.

I could write for another 10 pages, but the preceding paragraph describes my perspective and year-to-year practice for surviving humanity (both my own and others). The other aspect of my success has to do with appreciating what I have been blessed to have and that which I have been blessed to... not have; whether I wish and pray for it and get it or not. The other portion of my success has to do with relenting to the power, will and plan of the Creator. Putting all my reliance, hopes, fears, needs, and rewards for doing what's right into one Devine basket, is my idea of faith. So far it has worked just fine, fulfilling every aspect of my life.

The final, element of my success is the most important of all. It is being blessed by the One who gives out all blessings. My contribution to my own success is in submitting to the will of God and being content with God's provision. To be honest, it feels good to be free of the search for help, answers, purpose, and "The way." It feels good to stop searching for the answers so that I can start doing and living the answers. It's perspective and relief that is hard to communicate without sounding arrogant. Many have succumbed to arrogance because of their "Relationship with God." This defeats the purpose of the relationship, which is to be humble, to share that relationship, and to, at least, be a good example and benefit to all others whether they believe as you do or not. Basically, if my relationship with God causes happiness only for myself but division, disdain, and distance with regards to my relationships with humankind, then... I'M DOING IT WRONG!

Biography

Kamau Sullivan

Writer of Essays and Fiction & Network Engineer

email: straiff@hotmail.com

Kamau graduated from Indiana University. He taught Language Arts before becoming a Network Engineer. Kamau has written a ten-book work of fiction entitled "Children of Renaissance". He is currently recording the first book as an audiobook and has hopes in submitting both forms of the book to a publishing company later this year. Kamau hopes to host a podcast with which he can help address issues which effect the human condition. In the meantime, he has recorded five videos on YouTube: https://www.youtube.com/playlist?list=PLwb1kM_w1X0t MIeyezDliSekokJGLj0lO. Topics include:

1. Time to Give Back - helping the self appreciate and protect the self
2. Nurturing Hope - re-igniting the pilot light of hope within the heart and mind
3. Your Right to Mental Wellness - concepts to practical mental wellness
4. Anger the Destroyer - Exposing the sneaky path to anger

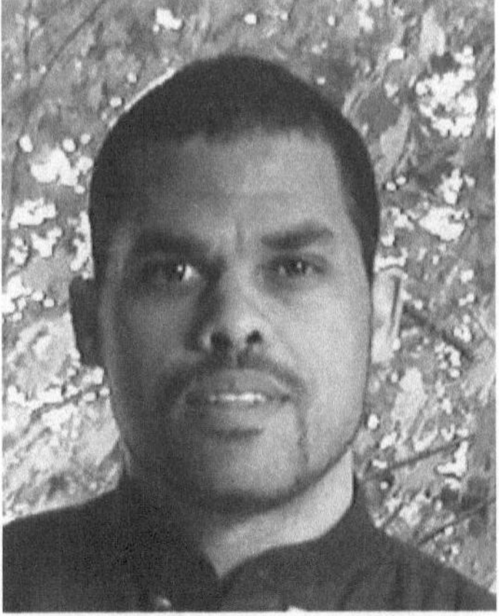

Chapter IV.

Crying Out

Boys don't cry.
That's what they said.
Stand up straight,
and comb your head.
What's wrong with you,
you're not like dad,
he was strong,
you're weak and sad?
I heard these words,
for years and years.
Why can't they see,
beyond my tears?
I cut myself,
to show my pain.
They just ignore,
the red blood stain.
I bite my arm,
and bang my head.
Please help me, please,
or I'll be dead.

Angela Washington

Chapter V.

He Heard My Cry for Help!

Dempris Gasque

"Do not conform to the pattern of this world but be transformed by the renewing of your mind. Then you will be able to test and approve what God's will is—his good, pleasing and perfect will." Romans 12:2

"Take me! God please just let me go. I don't want to live anymore. I'm tired. I'm tired because no matter how hard I try I'm never enough. I'm seen, but I've never been heard. I have a hole in my heart, and it hurts every single day.

I go to school and I see my peers and they talk about their dads. How their fathers spent time with them outside, how they went to a game, and mine just left me. Left me like I was an afterthought. I never really mattered and God if you could let someone come into my life, make me, and then abandon me like I was nothing then maybe I am nothing. And if that's the case, what's the point? I'm going to hell anyways. I try to control myself when I'm in church they say it's an abomination. I'm going to burn in hell FOREVER. For an attraction I didn't ask for, one I've never understood. I've questioned myself so many times, what's wrong with me and why I can't just focus on females. Something about a guy that I'm attracted to, like a moth to a flame since childhood, but it's forbidden. I didn't even know what sex was when I began to notice an attraction to the same sex. I was young, but it was the most natural thing to me. I didn't understand at that age that I would face so much backlash, distain, or even disgusted looks of disappointment. So please, TAKE ME.

I'd rather you just kill me now or let me be killed than live every day with a cloud over my head as if running from an eternity I can't fix. I wish I could just straighten up and be more masculine, that I dreamed of a wife and kids, but I keep thinking about my best friend. I'm Christian, I think, but can I be? There's no home for me. If I go to church I'll be judged, but it's frowned upon not to go. I keep replaying my death in my head, you watched me write my suicide note, you heard what my mother said. She'd never raise a gay son. So, what's left? Do I just cut myself? I tried the other day, but I don't like blood and that would take too long. I thought about shooting myself but with what gun? The quickest way seems to be a car accident, but how do I make sure I die? I don't want to live and wake up in a hospital then must do it all over again.

Why can't you just let me die? Send someone to rob me, let me get hit by a car, or shot walking from the school bus? Or get my mom to do it? She hates me anyways; she looks at me sometimes with such disappointment. I've prayed to you and asked you to fix me, make me straight, take away my attraction to people all together, just let me live alone. I won't do anything else.

I won't ever have sex. I'll even lie, blend in, settle down and get married to a female. Just take the pain and shame away. I try everything, I get nominated every year to be a White House ambassador, I'm an Honor Roll student, but I still get in trouble. Ridiculed for talking, but that's the only time other students talk to me. In class when they need help, other than that I'm the little black boy that might be gay.

They ask for my help, they know I know the answers, but they talk about me. They taunt me behind my back and call me all kind of names, then when I'm quiet my teachers make me help them. My teachers make me talk for participation, but it hurts all over again. Now I'm the kinda-sorta-might-be-gay-teacher's pet. Just let me go. You can't love me like the Bible says you do, you couldn't have sent a son to die for me, no man would come down and willingly die for someone who may be gay. There can't be a Jesus or God if you'd let your people suffer so much, killing themselves to be perfect.

I see and feel things. I can feel people's emotions, but it feels like I'm the only one that can. When we went to church last week, this little voice told me that the pastor used to be an alcoholic and I could see their whole life.

Am I broken? Is this normal or am I losing my mind? I hear voices and one told me when someone would die. Why is it that when I write I begin to see the characters I'm writing about? What the hell is wrong with me? Please. Please. Please! Just let me die, I don't understand, and I feel like I'm suffocating every day. I'm drowning, but no one can hear me and it's like I'm in the middle of the ocean and every time I think I'll finally die, that the pain of living like this will be over, I catch my breath and spit up water. I almost die or I think I do, but then you wake me up. You wake me up and make me start the day all over.

You hate me so much for my attraction that you'd wake me up and make me relive these moments again until I get it right. Can you at least teach me? Teach me how to "straighten" up. I wear baggy clothes already; I can learn to play sports too. Instead of reading this weekend I'll go play basketball. I'll play all day, but then I'll think of my dad again and the hole in my heart, the fact that you gave all my little cousins fathers and moms, but you said no not Dempris. He doesn't deserve it. He'll be ok. Skip over him.

My mom will ask if I'm okay, and I'll lie and say it's my allergies again. I have allergies but does she really believe me or does she just not wanna talk to me? Either way I didn't touch the food she cooked last night. I threw it in the trash. I moved some of the trash out the trash, folded the plate in half, then stuffed it down. Something about how she looks at me with disgust, I'm not eating that food. It might be poisoned. I stayed up late last night watching the door. I didn't want to see anymore demons, shadows, or wonder if she'll kill me in my sleep. I'm sure I sound crazy and we don't talk about it, but I look like my dad. And every time she looks at me, I think she sees him and gets angry all over again. So, I'm the kinda-sorta-might-be-gay-teacher's pet-mom's-greatest-disappointment-Gods-abomination.

Great! Just fucking great Dempris! What's wrong with me? What did I do wrong? God was it the one time I played with that baby doll or took one? I don't even like dolls, my cousins all had one, so I just wanted one. But I never liked girl toys or clothes. I just wanted to see why it was so much fun to them. But if that's why you made me gay only to label me with sin for an attraction when I'm not even having sex, why can't you just take me now? Just take me to hell now please. I don't wanna wait and fall in love with someone I could never be with, then must distance myself from my family. I love my family, but I see the way they look at me and talk about me too. I don't know how to keep loving myself in such a cruel world. I'm just a kid. Please. Please. Please just kill me. Matter of fact, I'll do it myself.

Tomorrow when I wake up. I'm tired, I'm ready to end this. How do you fix a boy that was born with a broken heart? I would pray, but you don't listen to people like me. We just burn in hell. Tell me what to do. I'm just tired and I don't know if I really want to die or if I just want the pain to stop. It just seems like pain is inevitable unless I stop breathing forever. At least then I'll know where I'll be instead of wondering every day and being too scared to live and too frightened to die. I guess I'm a coward. The truth in saying that seems to be as ugly as the blackness of my skin.

I'm tired of people asking me if I'm from Africa. I don't even know my dad and barely know my family history, but I'm supposed to know if I'm from Africa? Are they trying to say I look poor or dirty? Every time I've seen Africa, it's from a charity commercial needing donations. Do I look poor? I may be poor or maybe I've poured out my soul in my tears from so much crying, I look like I need help. But the ones asking are the same ones that talk so bad about me so why would I take the help? They must think I'm stupid. Stupid enough to allow them to see my insides, I can't be vulnerable, that makes me weak.

I'm a black southern boy. Why did you do this to me? Why did you create me? Please tell me why you made me and why I can't seem to love myself? I'm just so helpless, ugly, and broken. Will this ever change? A voice keeps telling me to pray, but I feel like prey. A weak mind, tempted flesh, displaced, and forgotten in a cruel world. I feel hopeless. I've already tried to take my life, unsuccessfully.

There seems to be nothing left. God, I don't know if you really exist, but if you do, I ask you to look after me. I've tried everything and everyone, but I'm tired. I'm too young to be tired, but I am. I'm tired of running feeling like I have no place here on Earth and that I'm unworthy of your glory. I'm tired of feeling like an afterthought or the remains of a broken or unused condom. I may not have experienced it, but I heard that there's more to life than this. I've heard of something called joy and I know I probably don't deserve it, but I'll ask for it anyways.

I don't know how to love myself, so I don't know how to love you, but I heard that you give grace and mercy. Allow me grace to understand why you created me because there must be more to my life than suffering. There must be a calling birthed out of all this pain, I may not be Shadrack, but I've been through the fire. I've been burnt, bruised, and battered, but I can't go another day feeling so empty, so miserable. I need you. I need you to hold me close to your heart and never let me go. I need you to wrap your arms around me and give me the love no one else can.

I need you to teach me how to be more like you. I don't want to be so broken, to be less of a man or to be so empty. Make me whole. Train me in the way that I shall go. I've sat in church all my life and I know I don't call on your name often, but I'm calling on it now. I've tried every resource, I've tried every suicidal attempt I could think of, I've came so close to death, the only thing left to do is to live. But I can't live like this. Give me a clean heart. Guide me with compassion and love. Forgive me because I don't think I'll ever be perfect, but if you'd just show me that you're real, I'd let you guide me by hand. Please God save me. Take me by the hand and show me how to live with the thorn in my side. Mold me into the person you have called me to be so that I may not always feel so empty. Fill me up with an outpour of your life. I've never experienced love, but I know it silences and heals pain. I just want to be able to look at myself and not cry. I'm tired of looking in the mirror and crying because of how dark and ugly I am, because my lips are so big, because I look like him or because I can't look at myself without seeing what others say about me.

I've heard people at church call you a potter or something? If that's the case, can you remold me? Just let me start fresh and wake up for just one day without thinking of killing myself or feeling hopeless. Just one day where I can just feel loved, instead of constant ridicule. Just one day of rest, I get so tired, but then scared to go to sleep. I have dreams I don't understand and then I wake up to a bitter world. God if you're real, please just hold me tonight. I don't remember what it's liked to be hugged, embraced, or warm. I just want to feel like everything will be okay. I feel like I'm expected to grow up so fast, but I can't keep up. I kill myself trying to please everyone else, I promise I won't be gay if you would just love me. No one else will. Not if they knew the truth. Why couldn't I be light skin or white? Born into a rich family so I could just buy stuff and be happy? I'd be happy if I were rich. And I could buy stuff that would change my dark skin. God please, why do I have to be so black? You can barely see me in photos. If you really exist, please just fix the hole in my heart. Teach me how to be okay with living because I know I'm too satisfied with the sound of death."

With tears down my eyes, I prayed. I prayed and prayed until my throat was dry and although I didn't have all the answers, I remembered Psalm 18:6. I cried and cried because I realized that Gods love was already bestowed upon me, I just hadn't accepted it. In my sadness I couldn't see through my tears. Not enough to see God's hand reaching out to guide and embrace me. Although I felt like absolutely nothing, I had to make a decision to seek God. I'd allowed people to determine what my life would be, but I needed to live long enough to understand why God didn't let me die on the day I tried to take my life. By faith I learned to understand. So, chin up king, God loved me with all my brokenness, and I know he loves you too!

The Bending Road That LED to My Recovery

1. Discipline- My ability to commit to my mental wellness was dependent upon my ability to set boundaries and develop daily practices that would help calm my anxiety and conquer my depression.

2. Accountability- Although discipline was extremely important, it meant nothing if I was unable to hold myself accountable. Although I cannot control others, I could learn to develop coping mechanisms and exercise healthy practices such as a Wellness Recovery Action Plan.

3. Honesty- One of the toughest things to do, I had to dig deep to realize I enabled people by allowing myself to be constantly disrespected. Feeling that I needed people because of their title or my fear of loneliness, I put others on a pedestal which was EXTREMELY toxic. Learn to be honest with yourself to replace bad habits with healthy wellness check-ins.

4. Forgiveness- It was easy for me to forgive others, my

Christian worldview required that I learn how to forgive those who hurt me but forgiving myself was nearly impossible. Because I was depressed and suicidal for YEARS, nearly a decade, I felt too ashamed to seek help and felt that I was weak. I had to learn to forgive myself for the self-inflicted harm and heartache I intentionally caused while self-sabotaging.

5. Inner Fulfillment- Self-doubt nearly crushed my spirit! Due to the fact that I always felt inadequate or less than because of my upbringing, belonging to a single parent, my attraction to the same sex, and competitive nature, I sought healing outside of myself. TOXIC relation, relationships, and even professional relationships. I developed unhealthy habits of clinging onto people that I knew couldn't positively serve me. BIG MISTAKE! I had to search within and become the person I needed.

6. Exercise-The clarity that comes with a healthy lifestyle is awe-striking! I started exercising for vain reasons, just being honest, however, along the way my doctor informed me of the importance of mental AND physical wellness and its influence on your overall health. Even if just 30 mins a day three times a week, exercise allowed me to heal.

7. Relationship- Now, I know I said I had been in some toxic relationships, BUT I had to sit myself down to determine what I needed, unapologetically. The National Alliance on Mental Illness further taught me how to maintain my mental and emotional health and became family to me. I also have accountability partners that are brutally honest and remind me to take care of myself and get adequate rest.

8. Prayer- While I am not here to change anyone's religion, I do know that prayer aided in my recovery process. Prayer activated purpose and allowed me to be led to my destiny. I found myself at peace and most able to heal when surrendering to God. I was not honest in most of my relationships due to fear, so prayer taught me how to live with conviction and made me realize I was worthy of help.

9. Aromatherapy- Eucalyptus, lavender, lemongrass etc. etc. etc. I love my diffuser and its oils. I have a diffuser, roll on body oil, and even therapeutic body oil I can apply after a shower. The healing properties are amazing and aromatherapy is fairly simple and easy to integrate into current wellness practices.

10. Cleansing- You are what you eat! Learning the need for freedom and rejecting the sense of burdening, I quickly realized that I did not want to feel heavy, spiritually, emotionally, or even physically. After my initial suicide attempt, I began to search for freedom of my mind and body. In doing so, I learned to change my eating habits and plan meals that were nourishing for longevity and even mental clarity.

Biography

Known widely for his community advocacy and passion for human rights, **Dempris Gasque** spends much of his time coordinating community events, cohosting a radio show on WIDU and developing initiatives to establish equitable solutions to ending institutional and systematic racism. The Certified Business Consultant and Expert Advisor is the CEO of The Mail Initiative, LLC., a consulting firm that offers business planning, legal services, and corporate printing solutions. Dempris Gasque also uses his experience as a National Alliance on Mental Illness and National Association for the Self-Employed Member, to promote personal and professional development on his blog. Gasque continues to share his story of triumph and truth with his unique writing style to inspire underrepresented populations in the hopes of building a future that learns to embrace people of color.

Chapter VI.

*Chapter Five is dedicated to my
older brother, whom is a
Decorated Army Veteran and an
Indiana Army Reservist that
passed by way of
Suicide September 2016.*

Salute SFC Randolph Davison, Jr.

*I love and miss you immensely.
Lil sis,
Venessa*

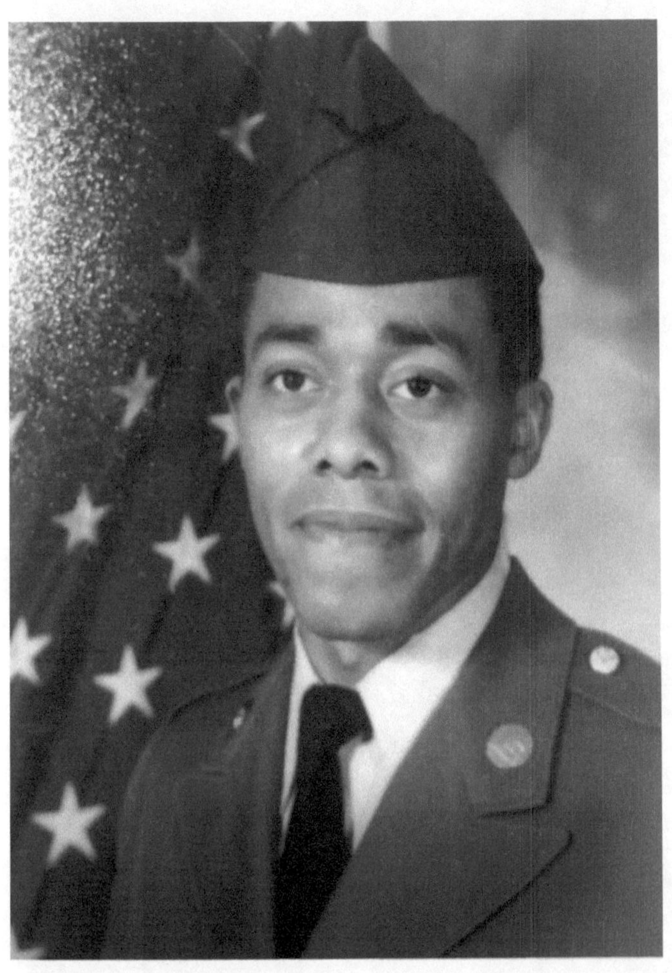

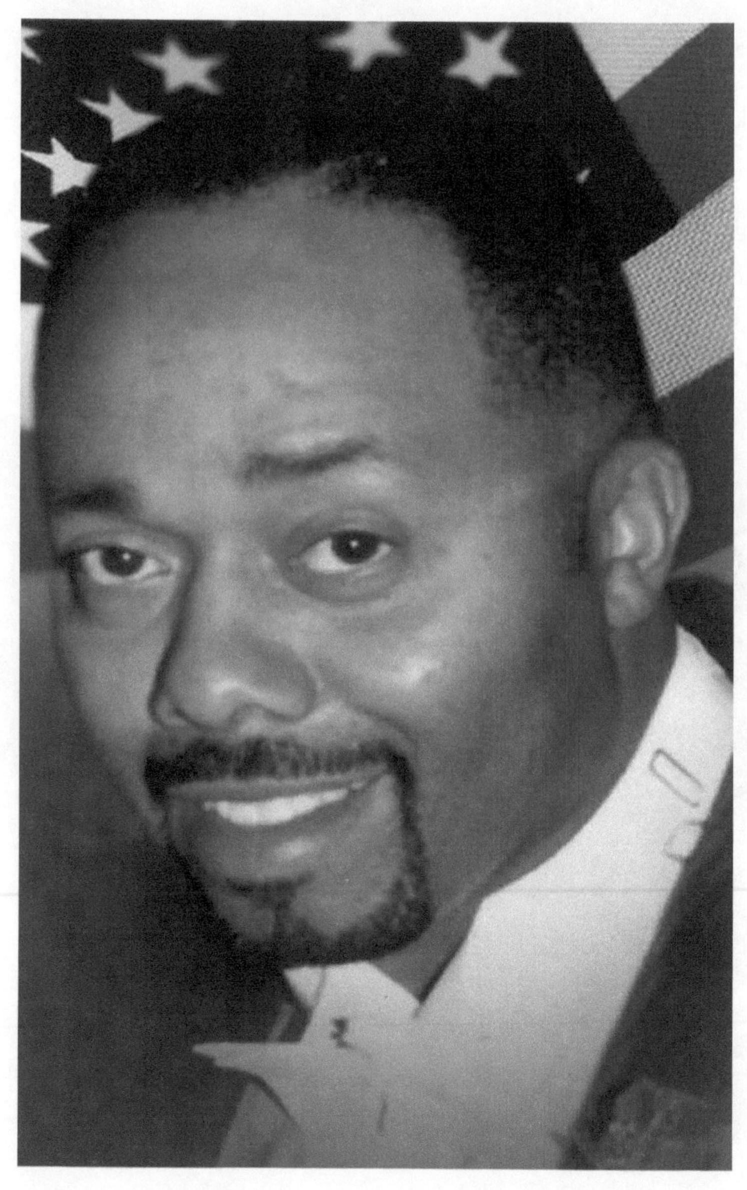

Reserved for

U.S. Army Veteran

SFC Davison

<UNTOLD STORY>

Reserved for

U.S. Army Veteran

SFC Davison

<UNTOLD STORY>

Chapter VII.

Function and Maintain

I'm a man and a father.

I'm a friend and a son.

I'm the one that keeps things going,

when the others go have fun.

I'm the one momma leans on,

when my siblings are around.

I'm the one my boss calls,

when his plane hits the ground.

I'm the one under pressure,

like the steam in a pot.

Everyone thinks I'm cool,

when inside I'm boiling hot.

I'm the one taking Xanax,

weekly talking out my pain.

I'm the one that knows with help,

I can function and maintain.

Angela Washington

Biography

The phenomenal poetic works of this Georgia peach, **Angela Washington**, are expressions of the heart, soul, everyday events, and once-in-a-life memories. She writes poems as if she is painting a picture. Each stanza is immersed in the emotions of a powerful moment. Angela is a poet gifted to tell stories that the world wants and needs to hear.

From a young age, Angela's had an artistic side that manifested itself from drawing in elementary school to playing drums in middle school. Ordained as a missionary at the age of twelve, Angela did what many middle schoolers didn't do-she traveled throughout central Florida sharing hope and inspiration. The poet, who received her Psychology B.A. from University of North Florida and Business B.S. from Jones Business College at Jacksonville skillfully combines her formal education, life experiences and natural leadership abilities to teach organizations that hope, improvement and achievement are only steps away.

Angela is a Multi-Award-Winning Author that has over 900 poems copyrighted at the Library of Congress. Many of her inspirational poems have been read by a global audience of the Steeple Award's Media Publication Magazine of the Year/2019, The Christian View Magazine issues June 2016 to September 2019 and other inspirational materials. For more information and booking inquiries contact Angela Washington at her website, www.angelofwords.com.

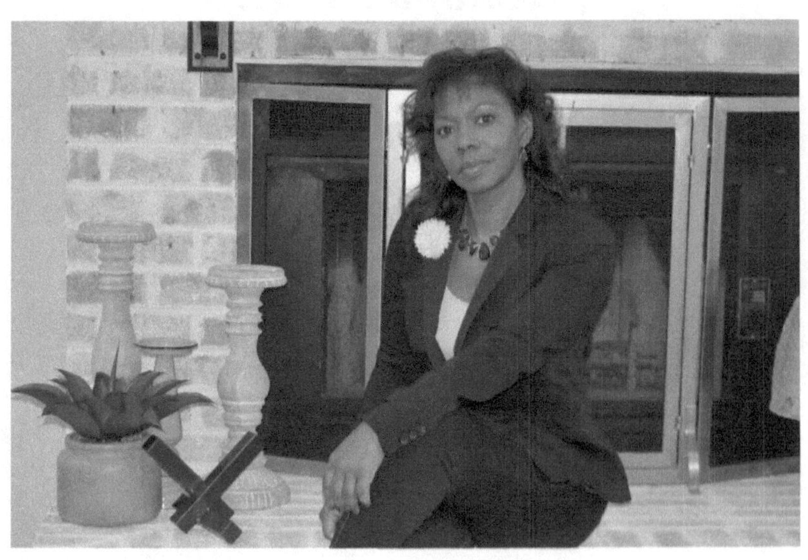

Chapter VIII.

Map to Mental Wellness Success: Dignity

John E. Sullivan, LCSW

I have a dream that my four little children will one day live in a nation where they will not be judged by the color of their skin, but by the content of their character.
— *Dr. Martin Luther King Jr.*

Overview

It is not by chance that way too many 'people of color' in our society, indeed the world over, struggle to view themselves as worthy and dignified. Part One of this essay relates occurrences during what I term the "Age of Un-enlightenment" that continue to negatively impact black and brown citizens of our planet. ***It is the ideological knee on their neck.***

The focus in this Series is on men, but that does not in any fashion suggest that these unpardonable events somehow left women unscathed. A discussion of the historical roots of ideologies of 'whiteness' and 'white supremacy' is crucial to understanding the origin of current notions of race and race relations. Perceptions arising in the Age of Reason continue to mar how we think about and act towards the overwhelming majority of peoples inhabiting the globe. The term 'non-white' is racist given that white people are a *minority* globally speaking. As such, it is more accurate that the white minority be labeled "people of non-color". It seems Dr. Frances Cress Welsing was the only person to understand this truism.

This writing begins with Dr. Oludamini Ogunnaike's insightful and informative account of the machinations of 17th to 19th century European philosophers and other intellectuals. Part Two is an expanded Map to Mental Wellness Success which is usually the last section of chapters in this Series. As such I have made it part of the title.

Part One

Origin of Bizarre Notions

What follows are highlights from A Conversation with Oludamini Ogunnaike in which he responded to the question, "Can we free our minds in a Post-Colonial world?" My commentary appears as italicized *Arial Narrow Font* within brackets [   ] . Let us ensue with his remarks.

We tend to think of modern education as a kind of neutral thing. [*He explains how the educational system imposed on colonial subjects was far from 'neutral'.*] We find that in the African context the colonialist were more so Britain and France and they were faced with how to govern so much land and so many people with only a few colonial officers. They decided the best way to gain and then maintain control of their colonial subjects was to mold young minds through 'education'.

The students were taught about themselves from the perspective of the colonizer. That is, from the outside. As a result, the youth developed a sort of double consciousness: what William Edward Burghardt Du Bois dubbed "a knowledge of self as other" [*The colonial masters institutionalized indoctrination under the guise of a so-called 'educational system' that gave birth to the bizarre notions which undermined any hope for the development of dignity among the youth. Oppressors and the oppressed still labor under these and other racist ideologies.*] For example, they were taught:

a. History (including their own) from a modern English perspective.
b. The myopic European version of 'true' knowledge and therefore 'true' intellect accompanied by an explanation of those amongst humanity who possess a higher level of both and those that do not.
c. That their ancestors were barbarians, uncivilized and lacked culture.

Interestingly, imperialistic tactics were not limited to 'Brown places.' The English attempted to do the same in Ireland where the Irish language was almost wiped out. [*That these people later gained acceptance points to the difference between being a victim of oppression as many white people are verses being a victim of oppression AND racism which is the lot in life of people of color.*]

White supremacy emerged from a shift in medieval enlightenment from endorsement of the Grand Chain of Being [*A hierarchical structure of all matter and life, thought in medieval Christianity to have been decreed by God. The chain starts with God and progresses downward to angels, humans, animals, plants, and minerals*] …this hierarchy was supplanted by one in which God was 'replaced' by man at the top of the chain. [*This sleight of hand in broad daylight occurred when during*] the Age of Enlightenment the concept known as the "super rational faculty of intellect (understanding)" was discarded. Supposedly this faculty enabled man to directly intuit God and higher levels of reality (i.e. Angels). At one time, this "super rational faculty" ranked higher than simple 'reason' and 'senses' as a means of 'knowing'. However, when it lost favor among philosophers and other intellectuals only reason and senses was left. [*This meant upper levels of the Great Chain of Being "went away" as well. And God was jettisoned from the hierarchy all together. The 19th century German philosopher, Friedrich Nietzsche, was emboldened to declare "God is dead".*]

So, who did that leave at the top the 'chain'? Man. And not man as a universal, but *white European rational man*. [*This last point cannot be over emphasized. This "We're-Number-One" mentality has been endorsed and nurtured from the onset of the Age of Enlightenment aka the Age of Reason in the 1600's to this very day. It continues to provide the demented 'rationale' for white supremacy. But wait, there's more. Additionally, this change at the top meant that what previously had been seen as worthy and thereby brought dignity to humans—the divine nature within humans—was replaced by the faculty of reason. Hence, the gloss 'Age of Reason'.*]

[Dr. Ogunnaike goes on to explain that] Reason becomes the full mark of humanity and only Western European man was considered 'fully rational'. Therefore, the only full (complete) human being. [*This racial narcissism was seen to play out in the United States Constitution where it was written, "enslaved blacks in a state would be counted as three-fifths of the number of white inhabitants of that state". It became easy to manipulate the wording of what came to be known as the "three-fifths clause" as a way to 'legitimize' treating African Americans as less than human.*]

[*From the point of view that white European man and not God was now at the 'top of the heap' as it were, it was a simple step to henceforth rank 'the other']* according to how close a particular racial/ethnic group is culturally and even in physical appearance to white European man.

So, Japanese were higher on the 'chain' than Chinese cause they look more like white people. Persians were defined as better than Arabs and Arabs better than Africans. [*And finally, Africans better than Negro Americans which is why the white owner of the liquor store in the predominately black neighborhood where I lived in St. Louis, always hired Africans instead of 'negroes' to work the cash register.*] W.E.B. Du Bois said, "The negro went from being viewed as a human being, but a heathen in the pre-Renaissance times, to after the Enlightenment being seen as subhuman." [*It is curious that the white folks, behind this historical farce considered themselves to be "enlightened" and "reasoned"! This begs the question: "***How long are people of color (the majority) going to be subjugated to the grandiose mentality of the minority on this planet?***"]

The Conversation with Dr. Oludamini Ogunnaike ends with these two points:

The hierarchy of angels in the traditional sacred Christian "Chain of Being" was replaced with a racial hierarchy.

Whiteness [*aka 'white privilege'*] was born as the *transcendence of race*. Not as one particular ethnic category amongst others. To be white is to transcend race.

I want to conclude with one last bit of commentary, appearing again within brackets.

[*Basically, white European males put themselves in place of God on the Grand Chain of Being. This point has been made numerous times for emphasis, it being key to this entire discourse. After discarding God, His Angels and Saints from the 'chain', white European philosophers and other intellectual movers and shakers provided their 'tribe' with the rationale for assuming the task of civilizing everyone else. The 'other' was, after all, further down the 'chain' which is where they must be since they were not fully human. This mischief gave birth to racist and imperialistic ideologies such the 'White Man's Burden' and 'Manifest Destiny'.*

In repeated instances the white minority among inhabitants of the planet operate as if they are the majority. As if their behavior is simply 'human nature'. As if what they say, think and do is 'the norm'! And herein lies prodigious trickery. For when 16th century Europeans replaced God with themselves at the pinnacle of the "Grand Chain of Being" it was not 'man as a universal'. Instead, white European man became THE universal.

The reader is asked to pause, re-read, and then ponder this last point.

This slyness is why in this nation, where white people will soon be the minority, the unemployment rate among white folks can be portrayed as THE "national unemployment rate". In my neighborhood referenced above, we had a saying, "Same game with a different name."]

Part Two

Map to Mental Wellness Success

My Map to Mental Wellness Success delineates how to cultivate and enrich personal worthiness and dignity and through this work begin to Recover from the calamity foisted on humanity spelled out in Part One.

Cultivation and Enrichment of Worth and Dignity –

The internal cultivation and enrichment of *worth* and *dignity* cannot be subject to or dependent upon how others view and attempt to define us. Criteria and definition of human worth and dignity must come from a Source that transcends humanity. The power to define a 'worthy and dignified' member of the human family does not rest with members of our family, except by default. In a 1964 presentation at the <u>Mary Hemingway Rees Memorial Lecture Series</u> sponsored by the World Federation for Mental Health, Mazhar Shah warned: "Having been given the freedom for a high purpose man cannot be left to be the law unto himself or otherwise he would try to equate even moral laws to personal ends." A variation of this is exactly what Dr. Oludamini Ogunnaike so eloquently explained.

The process of cultivation and enrichment leading to recovery begins by identifying Attributes of the Creator. Doing the work to reflect these Attributes and then to manifest them into our world promotes and instills dignity in a way that is profound and, equally important, lasting. So long as the source of attributes, qualities or character traits we seek to nurture within ourselves is other than that which transcends our horizontal plane of existence, we shall continue the futile exercise of replacing one reductionist approach to human relationships with still another. We will continue to labor under the modernist myth that change equals 'progress'.

The Attributes of the Creator are of a different order. They are *absolute*. The absolute Attribute of Justice, for example, means the Creator is in no way unjust to any part of creation. Humans are unique within creation in that we have the spiritual anatomy that enables us to 'reflect' Attributes of the Creator in a finite way. Furthermore, through our actions, we can manifest them in this world. One writer describes human beings as the 'cosmic bridge' from the Creator to this domain. The more of these Attributes we exemplify the more imbued we become with worth and dignity.

Readers who have already succumbed to what I refer to in other writing as 'the last taboo', may be experiencing uncomfortableness with references to the 'Creator'. The 'last taboo' is the one that makes it culturally prohibited (euphemistically referred to as 'politically incorrect') to speak of the Creator and things related to the Creator, i.e. the Attributes of the Creator. I call this prohibition the LAST taboo because when this subject matter is taboo, then what separates humans from other creatures cannot get oxygen. When those things which separate us—our unique relationship to and knowledge of our Creator are no longer valued— we forfeit our humanity.

Recovery

Humanity needs to Recover from the racist Eurocentric view of 'the other'. Readers who digest and seriously consider the ramifications of Dr. Ogunnaike's conversation have already begun this Recovery work. It starts by educating one's self about the origins of our group think regarding 'the other'.

We must replace 17th century criteria for 'ranking' our fellow human beings. Then we need to modify our behavior towards them which up to now has been rooted in an arbitrary and artificial hierarchy hailed as the 'Great Chain of Being'. The position and status ascribed to those viewed as 'less than' has been affixed to the extent that some among them feel it necessary to sacrifice their worth and dignity by imitating *white European man*: culturally, socially and in their appearance.

The reality is that the best among us is the one whose consciousness of the Creator is most perfectly reflected in his or her behavior. What is unique and even elegant about *this* measure, is it cannot be known by human beings. This means stratification systems contrived by human societies are counterfeit. These systems are in no way related to the true worth and dignity of humankind.

Application of Map

The more committed one is to reflecting Attributes of the Creator, the more they reap the fruit of self-worth and dignity.

Here are examples of how eight Attributes/Qualities/Powers of the Creator can be reflected and then manifested in the world.

Let's begin with the Attribute of **Ruler** and the power of Ruling that comes with it. A person shares in this Attribute when he or she rules their own self. If we consider the *self* to be a 'kingdom', we can say our soldiers in this endeavor consists of our appetites, the emotion of anger and our affections (likings, preferences). Our subjects are our feet, hands, tongue, stomach, eyes, ears, and genitals. When we take responsibility for and rule these soldiers and subjects instead of being ruled by them, we reflect this Attribute of the Creator in a finite manner.

The Attributes (Powers) of *Abasing* and *Exalting* are reflected and then manifested when someone abases falsehood while at the same time exalts and supports truth. Abasing falsehood takes place on three levels. The most elevated level is to act against it. Another lofty level is speaking and/or writing against lies and misinformation when it first rears its ugly head. Finally, one can refuse to embrace prevailing propaganda. There are times and circumstances when the latter is all we can do.

Certainly, *Justice* is an Attribute of the Creator in sore need to be reflected in us and manifested in society. Individuals operate from the position of justice when their anger, passions and caprice are subservient to reason.

Patience as a Power/Quality/Attribute of the Creator is reflected in the human being who combines being patient with perseverance. This is an excellent definition of the quality of resilience so important to mental health. Being patience should not be confused with submissiveness. Patient perseverance requires experience, practice, and Guidance to oppose impulses of passion and anger.

It can be said that an individual reflects and then manifests this quality when two opposing motives contend for attention and subsequent action and that individual is able to repel the impulse leading to rashness and haste.

Total Awareness as an Attribute of the Creator speaks to a level of consciousness that human beings could never obtain. However, one who is aware of their *lower self* and its deceit, propensity for self-delusion and ruses is said to be aware. Cultivation and enrichment of this attribute enables one to guard against the lower self, adopting a watchful vigilance over it. However, when one actively opposes the guiles and promptings of his or her lower nature, that person has gone beyond mere reflection to an observable manifestation of this attribute.

Another quality of the Creator is **Majesty**. Human beings who reflect Majesty are deemed beautiful and majestic in the *true* sense of these words. *Their sense of worth and dignity heightens exponentially*! Their character traits become appealing and attractive so as to give pleasure to the faculty of discernment in others.

Reflection of the Attribute of Majesty requires, first of all, understanding that exterior beauty is of lesser worth. People who focus on the *interior* qualities of their fellow human beings have an interesting feature about them. They not only exhibit care and concern towards another person, their interest in that person goes even further. As such, they often ask that person how the people *around them* are faring as well. In other words, they want to know the affect this person is having on those in this person's sphere. This is taking care and concern for others to a whole new level.

As these examples illustrate, the process of reflection and then manifestation is not complex. It is remarkably simple and easy. Consider the Attribute of the Creator, **Loving Kindness**. It finds expression when the venerable 'Golden Rule' is valued enough to be practiced.

Biography

John E. Sullivan, MSW, LCSW. Retired. MSW 1971 University of Missouri. Adjunct Professor University of Indianapolis 26 years and Psychotherapist 44 years. Listed in <u>Who's Who</u>: <u>American Muslim Resource Directory 1994</u>. Director of Department of Correctional Facilities with the <u>Islamic Teaching Center of North America</u>.

Domestic and International Lectures/Presentations: Panel Member <u>C-Span</u>: "Muslim Families in America". Annual lectures <u>Indiana University Medical School of Bioethics</u>: "Considerations When Interacting with Muslim Patients and their Families." Presenter at <u>First World Symposium on Psychology and Islam</u> College of Education Riyad and <u>First Symposium on Islam and Psychology in America</u>. St. Louis University. Lectures on Islam and Psychology <u>Women's College in Omdurman</u>, <u>Sudan</u>. New Delhi <u>Islamic Institute of Islamic Studies</u> and the <u>University of Khartoum</u> – Sudan. Award Winning Author – "The Voices Behind Mental Illness

Publications:

Most Recent Article: "Preliminary Report on a Spiritually Based PTSD Intervention for Military Veterans." <u>Community Mental Health Journal</u>. Vol. 55, No. 5. 22 June 2019. Past publications include: Contribution to several Textbooks University of Indianapolis Press.

<u>Subhuman Behavior</u>. Amazon Books. Com

Biography Con't.

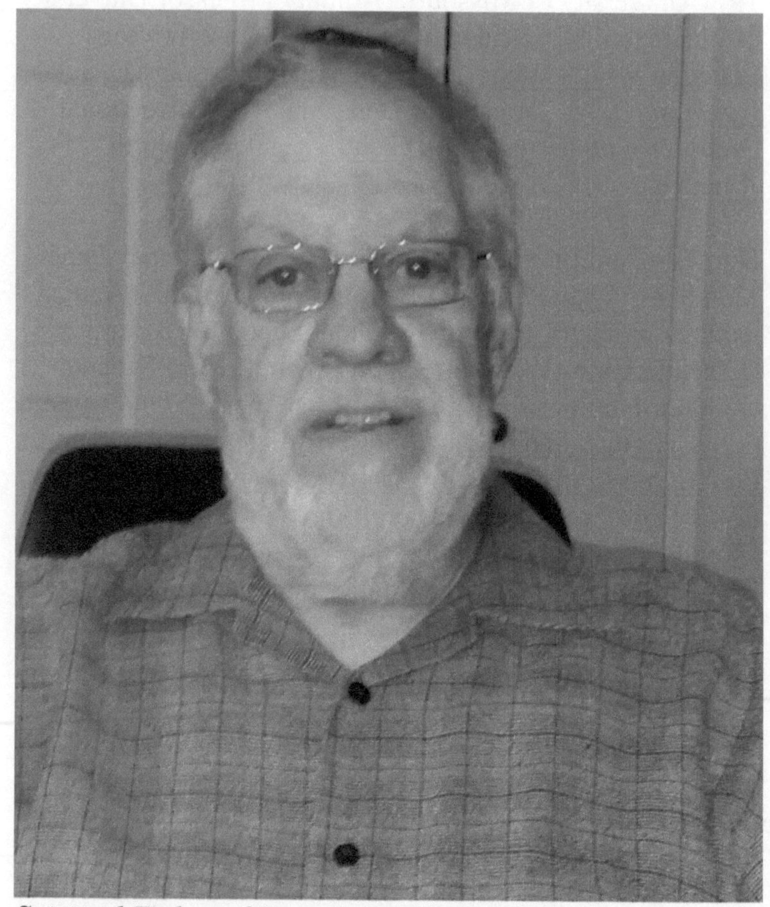

Spiritual Father of Venessa D. Abram

Chapter IX.

Mental Illness in the Family and My SDPPP Experience

Aaron Ballantyne

But my God shall supply all your need according to his riches in glory through Christ Jesus. Philippians 4:19

One of my most memorable experiences with mental illness was during a visit to my extended family.

While I knew this family member suffered from Schizophrenia, I didn't quite know at the time how it affects individuals who suffer from it or the extent to which it can impact their behaviour, so when that dear family member had an episode out in the street, I didn't know what to make of it or what to do.

Curse words were said, things were thrown and I sat in silence and bewilderment as my dear family member approached the house, grateful this energy wasn't directed at me or the fellow family member who sat beside me, also in silence.

However, following that experience, it has shed some light on a few things. As there have been episodes since then, to which I have been witness, I have learnt that mental illness, especially Schizophrenia, can affect individuals in various ways.

I've also seen the value of balancing how you treat someone with mental illness, meaning, not pitying them, or making them feel less than human or less deserving of love, while also not pretending they don't have a mental illness. It has also cultivated in me a deeper appreciation for

anyone suffering from mental illness, an appreciation
which has been taken to the next level ever since I joined
the SDPPP team.

Tasked with sending out SDPPP's monthly newsletters, I
was required to conduct research on various mental
illnesses in order to provide relevant, relatable and current
information to engage readers. It was while conducting this
research that my eyes were not only opened to the
prevalence of various mental illnesses, but also their
varying impacts and how they have affected the lives of
those who have them as well as their families and
caregivers.

This research and the findings which were unearthed
compelled me to become more detailed and dedicated to
providing helpful resources, information, and reassuring
inserts of encouragement to our readers.

When aligned with the overall mission of SDPPP and the
events, endeavors, efforts, causes and initiatives taken to
exact real change in the area of mental illness and health, it
really puts into perspective just how important awareness
and more importantly, support is for such a cause.

Biography

Aaron Ballantyne is a 24-year-old Freelance Writer who joined the *Self-Discovery PPP Team* in October 2018. Since then, he has undertaken a number of responsibilities and used his writing skills to help us with our mission to eradicate suicide. Today, he continues to use his talents to spread invaluable information on mental illness and shares his experience with us to encourage others and raise awareness.

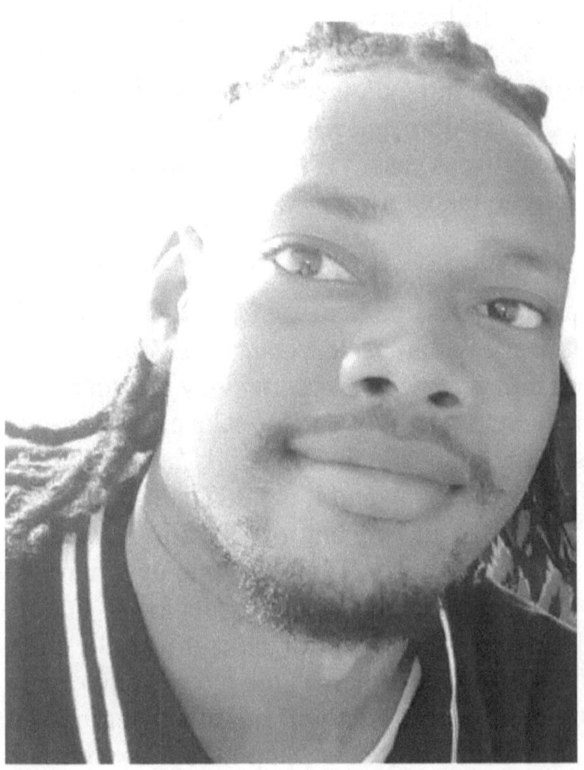

Chapter X.

Powerhouse of Peace

Bernard Davis, Jr.

The last shall be first, and the first last:
for many be called but few chosen.
Matthew 20:16

Growing up, all I ever cared about was making people smile. I would light up like a Christmas tree anytime I was able to bring a smile to others. Knowing the limits of happiness is wisdom and responsibility. I have learned the importance Just as easy it is to give someone happiness it just as easy to take it away.

 Knowing what makes someone happy is a fit and I look at happiness as a blessing because I had difficulties when being at peace with myself when I was younger. I always expected things to be in a specific way or order for things to work or for a positive result to take effect. I used to love making fresh lemonade for the family because my auntie made it a specific way and it would taste special every time, full of love and joy but it was from the heart. Going to buy lemonade. It always cheered me up when I was felt down, and I knew I had to learn the recipe so that if she needed me to make it, I would make it just like she would. She would also tell me don't give it to no one else or drink it all at one time because I will miss the happiness behind it. My aunt also said, "Your happiness is everything and if someone knew what made you smile or laugh, they would try and take it away from you. I would get so happy after a glass of cold lemonade and it was something my aunt would see, and she made sure to make it the same way every time for me.

As I got older, I started understanding the essence of my happiness and peace and how it can play apart of my health holistically, and it is something I kept with me moving forward as I grow into a young man. When I became 18-years old, I had a friend who had issues with self-confidence and would make others feel bad about themselves because he didn't have a personal connection with himself. Once I encountered that spirit, I automatically thought about my aunt and her lemonade and I decided to give him a few ideas on how to stay confident in situations that are out of our comfort zones. He was thrilled with what I shared with him, and I can truly see the difference it made after our conversation.

The next time we crossed one another's path, he mentioned he started using the technique in a negative manner to gain confidence over the people in the uncomfortable situation, instead of himself, and that even brought my energy down seeing something that's meant for good. I felt I had let my aunt, friend and myself and I confronted him about the situation. Luckily, I was able to get on a genuine page with him to help him understand buy when I first came across the situation my stomach flipped. I could only think about me being happy about my aunt's love, but I never thought about how someone else would feel in a similar station of self-happiness and peace is important to me. Going forward with life and my journey and I am grateful to be able to understand the value of it all.

Map to Mental Wellness Success

Knowing self being able to understand yourself in different environments.

Knowing the value of your platform understand the difference between yourself and something that has a connection you and your inner spirit.

Meditation - Learning how to process the different energy on a daily basis and learning how to keep it balanced.

Self-confidence - Being able to keep your energy/ideal character consistent to anything you are doing or going through.

Loyalty to the soul understanding the value of who your inner person is and learning how to reshape the form your spirit while keeping the same Aura/Peace.

Consistency - Learning how to keep a firm a solid connection with God and your spirit.

Biography

Bernard Davis, Jr., an Indiana Native, still resides in Gary, IN. Bernard is a Co- Author in the Book of Men and Mental Illness, and is an Andrean Highschool Graduate, who is dedicated to normalizing talking about mental health after experiencing a loss of a close friend from gun violence amongst men and their families-which Bernard has experienced with his friend back in 2019.

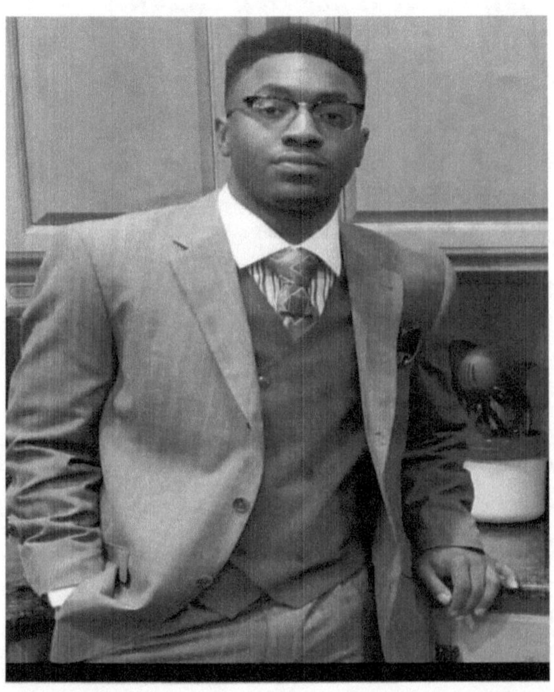

Chapter XI.

The End of A Cycle

Anthony L. Abram, Jr.

**"*For Generations we've been dealt
bad hands with bad plans" Kendrick Lamar
(Song: Nipsey Hussle- Dedication)***

Prior to 2015 and experiencing the stillbirth of my son due to pregnancy complications, I've been dealing with mental illness my whole life. Unbeknownst to me in my eyes growing up people who suffered from mental illness were— on drugs or homeless. Discussing mental health and getting educated on mental health was taboo. As a kid, every time a police car rode passed, I would hide. Looking back now, I thought that was normal. However, that was a sign of fear from all the traumatic stories I'd hear about the bad things police did to us.

Even today as a twenty-seven-year-old black male, while driving I get nervous when the police is behind me. Knowing I didn't commit any crimes I still begin to glare into each of my mirrors to make sure the officer hasn't turned their lights on— all while my heart is racing. PTSD (Post-Traumatic Stress Disorder) like symptoms has been caused from experiencing race-based stress and trauma frequently. Caused by a single event, racial stress is ongoing, pervasive, generationally transmitted, and affects both individuals and collective communities. All the videos on social media of the police killing those who look like me are examples of racial trauma. Systemic racism has its hands deeply rooted into the economic prospects, mental well-being, physical health, and daily lives of black people— and black children have always been watching and experiencing it.

Nevertheless, trying to seek mental health resources within the black community, we are still facing racial disparities. Compared to our white counterparts, we have less access to mental health services and the services we do have are more likely to end prematurely. There we are again stuck battling our problems on a daily basis without the proper treatment. Sadly enough for some African Americans their first encounter with mental health treatment is in the criminal justice system. Nearly 15% of men and 30% of women booked into jails have a serious mental health condition, according to the National Alliance on Mental Health. Once they're freed, housing and jobs are harder to come about. Without the proper treatment they're back to square one doing what will lead them back to jail.

At this stage you're probably wondering how this is affecting me mentally. Well it's affecting all of us. Most of us were born into these traumatic situations. To think I would have had a four-year-old son in this world today is mind boggling. He would've had so many questions on everything that's going on today. My only thought after I would have given him the honest truth and taught him not to have toxic masculinity—how would I have protected him? How will I protect my future children? How will I prevent my future daughter from going missing due to sex traffickers? Only thing we can do is keep God first and teach them how to survive. Educate them on their rights, black history, the importance of knowing who their voting for, and mental health. Ensuring we talk about mental health regularly. The things I didn't know about growing up, I can now educate my children on because now I know. That's how I will begin ending the generational cycles with my future family.

In the meantime, during this pandemic and all the fighting for justice and a new reform, I'll continue to find a peace of mind for myself. I encourage you all to unplug from the news and social media as well. All of this has been emotionally and mentally draining. Most of us have been in the house for months now, we still have to take a mental health day or two. Continue to invest in your mental health.

Biography

Anthony Abram Jr, an Indiana native, now resides in Atlanta, GA. Anthony is an Bestseller Author in the 'Series 3: The Mind Is A Terrible Thing To Waste, speaker for National Alliance of Mental Health, and Founder of Living Always Inc. Living Always Inc. is dedicated to normalizing talking about mental health after experiencing a pregnancy or infant loss amongst men and their families— which Anthony experienced with his son stillbirth back in 2015. Through Living Always Inc is the way that Anthony continues his son's Legacy forward.

Follow us on Twitter, Facebook, and Instagram:
@LivingAlwaysInc   Website: www.livingalways.org

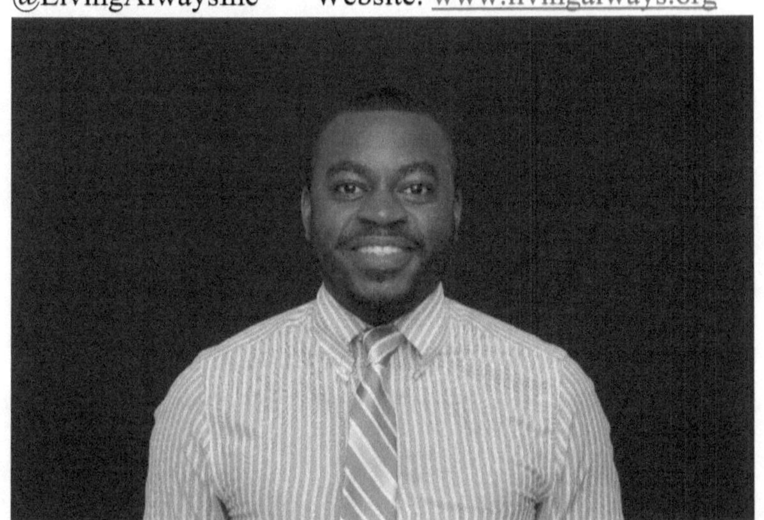

Chapter XII.

Recovering the Wreckage

Shane Foster

"My grace is sufficient for you, for my power is made perfect in weakness." 2 Corinthians 12:9

By the grace of God, the man writing to you today is doing just that, recovering. I am recovering from a multitude of challenges including childhood trauma, sexual abuse, substance use disorder, sex trafficking, organized crime, institutions, and a range of mental health challenges that come with a past like this.

From an early age, I realized that I was not like the other kids. A social reject. Apart from being different, my childhood was riddled with trauma. You see, struggle and trauma were something I inherited, but so was strength and perseverance. My mother, practically a child herself while raising my siblings and I, had been dealt a tough hand as well. Sexual abuse, neglect, abandonment, rape, alcoholism, domestic violence, and her own mental health challenges were just a few of the cards she was dealt. Looking back, I now understand what an amazingly strong beautiful women she was, and what a tremendous job she did.

A mom can always recognize her child's struggle with sexuality way before the child even has a clue. I was so lucky to have her to love and support me through finding and accepting myself. Unfortunately, a mother's acceptance isn't always enough.

By the age of twelve I realized that being a rebel, sneaking out and hanging with older kids, would get me the social acceptance I needed. This won me the girlfriend and social stamina I needed to boost me into my teen years. Little did I know that even this would come with a price. At fourteen, I was admitted into my first Mental Health facility for bi-polar disorder, manic depression, and suicidal tendencies. While gaining the social acceptance I felt so desperate for, I had lost personal acceptance in finding my true self. My life had become a lie.

I eventually found a way to explore my sexuality through chatrooms and phone sex lines. By seventeen, I had ignorantly decided that I had a hustle. These lines of communication had opened the door to a world of predators in search for guys like me. Guys who struggled with their identity, social and family rejection. Guys who were numbing the pain to accept who they were. Guys searching for a father figure. Guys desperate to make a few bucks. I was every predators dream.

These encounters lead me into some life changing experiences. I had met and built relationships all over the country ranging from Los Angeles porn producers to New York mobsters. I soon found myself as the center of a sex trafficking ring. Pulling guys like myself into various paid exchanges for sex. This connected me in some powerful ways and went on for fifteen years. This lifestyle had consequences though. I was way too young to have access to that type of money. Millions literally. Through the reckless generosity my social life grew, as did my drug habits. I had met some extremely wealthy men that were business savvy, and more than eager to show me their financial abilities.

I found myself living like a Rockstar. Multimillion-dollar homes, endless shopping sprees, expensive restaurants, and the finest of Hotels. With this came the endless supply of drugs. At first it was just cocaine, but eventually grew into the designer "circuit drugs" that swept Atlanta's gay culture. Ecstasy, GHB, Ketamine, and Methamphetamines soon became a daily part of my existence. My friends and I would spend days and sometimes weeks on our escapades.

This would become a problem for me. The drugs inevitably began taking control, causing me to lose control. Drug induced psychosis would grip me causing me to question my sanity. Countless times I would wake up from drug overdoses, confused and disoriented unsure of who or where I was. Paranoia and schizophrenia became a daily part of my life. I was robbing myself and hurting everyone around me. My lack of control caused me to rage out against people I loved. I needed help.

I was no stranger to the word help and what it consisted of. And I was not afraid to ask for it. I was afraid, horrified even, of losing my place in the lives of my investors. I was aware of how easily it would be to replace me. I was also aware of my having outgrown the criteria looking to be filled from previous relationships. These men were attracted to guys who were "barely legal" I was well into my late 20's. I had become extremely dependent on these relationships to afford the life I had created, regardless of how reckless or dangerous it had gotten.

I agreed to go into treatment. I had an open probation case, I had to be mandated for it to be approved by the felony probation department. I agreed. My family raised the money, and I went into residential treatment. Unfortunately, not all residential programs are clean, safe places. I kept my head down and attended meetings and tried to avoid the others in the program because it became clear that they were not all clean. The majority were just there to keep from going to jail. I found a local church and dug in. At least for as long as I could.

Four months into the program, I lost my job. I was struggling, and so was my family. Under the financial pressure of it all, I ended up leaving the program and using. This led to a violation of the felony probation case. The state ended up pulling it all and sending me to prison. This time I got lucky, after classification -I went to a ninety-day bootcamp and came home on parole.

I moved into the home of the New York mobster that had shamelessly fallen in love with me from the chatlines. This man would become known as my "god-father". His multimillion-dollar home was incredible. We both understood the reciprocity that formed our relationship. Although, old enough to be my father, the amount of generosity and encouragement I felt there would carry me through for years. I began being groomed for my career as a loan shark. We started with one store, a payday advance. I was loaning thousands of dollars out with 30% interest on seven day inclement. This went on for close to a year, until Georgia passed the law banning payday advance, so we then moved into doing title pawns. Through the title pawn industry, we built a sixteen-store empire, that eventually leads into me serving eight years in custody of the state.

In 2005 I had to be clean, so I began seeking medical help. I saw doctors, psychiatrist, hypnotherapist, and religious leaders from all over the state. Nothing seemed to help. During this insanely difficult time, through bloodwork being done by my physician, I learnt that I was HIV positive. My world came crashing down around me. Flashes of watching my uncle die from AIDS in the 80's haunted my sleep. I watched my family and loved ones grieve me as if I were already dead. My life felt as if it was over. My drug use hit new levels. I began injecting meth, pushing my spirit from its temple, leaving nothing but the flesh to guide my way. I began overdosing and self-destructing. I was angry at everyone. My temper raged right alongside of my diagnosis.

Soon my legal issues would catch up to me. I bounced all over Georgia serving a total of eight years in prison. Most of them in mental health facilities due to my background. Through this time, I would be exposed to a multitude of traumatic experiences. Violence, drugs, neglect, gang activity and even sexual assault were a part of the daily lives of the men inside these camps. I was put on a work detail, level five mental health dorm orderly. This detail consisted of helping these inmates maintain daily routines like housekeeping, hygiene, and mealtimes. Most of these guys were so sedated on medications, that even their most basic functions were impaired. I drew close to God, and he pulled me through.

My godfather was smart, while he sent me money, he used this time to put distance between us. By the time my sentence was served, I had lost my entire immediate circle. My mom to COPD and lung cancer, my biological father to a drug overdose, and several friends and cousins to drug related deaths. I came home to nothing or no one. I was lost. All the expensive habits and luxuries were like they never existed. I was left with nowhere to turn. My cries for help, went unheard. My burden was my problem. All the friends and acquaintances I had acquired left when the money did. I became suicidal as well as homicidal. I wanted everyone to feel the pain I was forced to endure. I was in a spiritual battle and hopelessly losing.

I was doing whatever to survive. I caught multiple new charges ranging from petty shoplifting to possession of methamphetamines. In my first attempt to resolve my legal issues I accepted banishment from the state on a felony drug charge, However, the remaining charges prevented me from leaving. I had to turn myself in and devise a new plan. Everyone kept suggesting Drug Court. I was not trying to hear it. I had been jerked around by the state enough. I was sure that it was a set up for failure. But something had to be done.

Finally, I decided to pray on it. Maybe this was the answer God decided to give me. If I set my mind to it, and trusted God to lead me, maybe, just maybe it would work. So, after contemplating it for several days I decided to try them with it. I wrote my public defender and asked for a sentence modification, in exchange for my participation in the Adult Felony Drug Court Program. What did I have to lose at this point? Sure enough, my public defender shows up to visit me at the county jail. He thought they would go for it.

In the blink of an eye, I was before the team answering questions about why I should be a candidate. Within a matter of days, I was released with orders to report to my case manager. It was bittersweet. The program seemed impossible at first. People were failing left and right. The things they were asking us to do were incredibly difficult. No contact with convicted felons, attend classes, hold a job, random screens, go to meetings, and bi-monthly court appearances were a lot. Overwhelming would be an understatement.

I kept my head down and did what they asked. I returned to church and got baptized. This would signify my rebirth to a new way of living. I worked an honest program. I found a sponsor and started doing step work. Six months in I started doing giveback projects. At least one was required to graduate. I created a community partnership between our court district and my church. This would upgrade treatment housing for three counties of Accountability Court programs. It afforded them room for expansion and several amenities like internet access, food bank access, nursery access and staff offices. It would also bring my church a substantial income.

The following summer we lost one of our youngest participants to an overdose. This jarred participants and staff alike. I co-hosted an overdose awareness ceremony, sharing on behalf of the family of our lost participant. We had a candle lighting ceremony allowing families from the community share on their loss and the impacts it had on them. We also had guest speakers raising awareness on statistics, prevention, and community supports. It was here that I knew that I had a calling on my life.

In February of 2020, I was accepted into the CPS Project. Through this project, I would become certified to use my lived experience in mental health recovery to coach and mentor others on their journey, I now mentor participants in both felony drug court and treatment court with plans to facilitate groups in the near future. I am also an advanced Achology Life Coach.

I'm a graduate from the Respect Institute, an organization that trains and promotes us to share our stories publicly in hopes of helping others. I have spoken several places throughout the state, to stake holders and peers alike, sharing my story of resilience and recovery.

I plan to continue my career in recovery. I am working my way into earning my CARES Certification (Certified Addiction Recovery Empowerment Specialist) and have plans to get involved with forensic mentoring, which will allow me to mentor state inmates looking to reenter society. My passion goal is to own my own line of transitional housing, providing men reentering society with safe stable housing in their own attempts to recover from institutions and hardships. From my own experience, I understand firsthand how challenging this can be.

This makes fifteen years I have lived with HIV. I'm happy to report that my virus is undetectable, and my immune system is operating at full capacity. Seeing a physician and taking only one pill a day, I can no longer transmit the virus to other people in any way. Glory be to God! I am learning to share about this virus openly. Speaking publicly about this gives hope to others who find shame in the stigma. The same goes for my recovery from sex trafficking. This trade is no longer only affecting females. Our teenage boys, and young men are being extorted and taken advantage of right alongside of our country's women. The impact this trade has can be overwhelming and extremely difficult to survive. However, recovery from this is also possible.

I am an active member in both the community and my church. I am beyond grateful for the direction God has led me in. It has become clear to me that I am on my Devine path. I no longer crave riches or the things that it brings. Now, I only want to return to the fire that had refined me almost to the point of death and save others burning as I did. I strive to draw closer to my savior and this divine path I have been given. Making gratitude my forefront is one of my greatest accomplishments.

Recovery is real. The light at the end of the tunnel is real. Reach for it. Be true to yourself. Don't give up on your dreams. It's never too late to reinvent yourself. Trusting God can be difficult and extremely uncomfortable at times, scary even. But if you can find it in yourself to do just that, trust God, his grace and mercy will lead the way. I have been turned into a living testament that miracles happen, and his promises are all true. With God, nothing is impossible.

Map to Mental Wellness Success

Throughout my journey *God* has always been my "go to" source for guidance and peace. Some of my earliest memories are my memories of childhood prayers. During my prison sentence, ***I kept notebook after notebook of prayer journals. These journals contained drawings, thoughts, prayers, and scripture***.

Narcotics Anonymous also became a part of my life at an early age. Sponsorship and working the steps afforded me the comprehension and spiritual awakening that I needed. Socializing with likeminded people was necessary, they genuinely loved me when I was unable to love myself.

The drug court's intensive treatment consisted of classes in anger management, moral recognition, cognitive behavior, and prime solutions helped rewire my thought process concerning my choices and actions. Coupled with hours of trauma therapy that aided in the unpacking and organizing traumatic occurrences and damage that got stuffed away during my efforts to forget and just survive.

Adult Children of Alcoholics and Dysfunctional Families has given me a psychological approach to reparenting myself that has served most effective. The step work and literature involved with this support group worked miracles as I was taught to recognize and forgive both myself and my parents for the hurt and pain I was forced to endure as a child in a dysfunctional home. This meeting will forever be a favorite of mine.

Taking full advantage of opportunities offered by the Georgia Mental Health Consumer Network like The CPS Project, and The Respect Institute gave me new light at the end of an otherwise dark tunnel. Through them, my struggles became strengths. The things society had previously penalized me for, were turned into credentials recognizing that the education life had given me was one that money could not buy.

I also make **self-care a top priority**. For me, that consist of restful sleep, alone time, prayer, meditation, as well as time with friends and family. Fine restaurants and shopping are a favorite past time. *My spiritual walk and involvement with the church* has been a constant support and reminder that God is always with me.

Everyone's recovery has its own path. No two journeys are the same. Now when I look at my recovery, I no longer see a hostile hopeless world. Instead I see a divine appointment in which I have taken my first steps into a destiny that gives my struggles cause and purpose.

Biography

Shane Foster is a Georgia boy through and through. He has overcome a multitude of challenges throughout his life. Rather than letting his struggles define him, he has chosen to take on a spirit of refinement. An Advanced Achology Life Coach, Mental Health Peer Specialist, and Public Speaker, Shane mentors' participants in both Adult Felony Drug Court and Treatment Court. Sharing his story publicly has given a voice to defeating a range of stigmas faced daily throughout our country. As an active member of his recovery community, he has taken his leadership ability and put it towards the greater good of society by doing successful projects that raise awareness, strengthen recovery ties, and promote community support. He recently accepted the role of Executive Director on the chair board for SDP3 and is anxiously anticipating what his future holds. Shane considers his path one of divine appointment.

Contact Shane Foster at: chair@sd-ppp.com

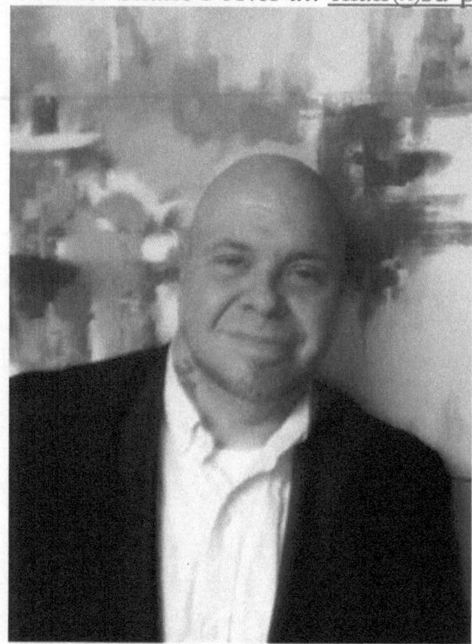

Chapter XIII

Man Down: Father Gone
Anais Nin

Dr. William "Flip" Clay

The human father has to be confronted and recognized as human, a man who created a child and
~ then, by his absence,
left the child fatherless and then Godless.

One of the greatest challenges facing young children today is growing up fatherless. There is no question that children who grow up in fatherless homes have a much greater risk of major challenges in life than those who grow up with a father at home. We might want to believe otherwise, and sometimes political correctness causes us to want to think otherwise, but the truth is, fathers' matter. In the United States, there are 9 million Black families, and the divorce rate is around 50%. Furthermore, in the Black family today, at least 63% of boys are raised by single mothers (4).

Early research portrayed African American fathers as generally absent or uninvolved in their children's lives (5). In contrast, more recent findings on African American fathers paint a different picture. This research shows that African American fathers, across socioeconomic and residency statuses, are involved with and interested in their children and can be nurturing and sensitive to their needs (6). Studies of resident fathers show that compared to White fathers, African Americans spend equivalent time in direct activities with their children and monitor their children more (7). Other, more nuanced findings show that fathers spend less time with their children during the week than during the weekend, and Black fathers have been found to spend more time on weekends relative to White fathers (7). The total amount of time spent with children and how it's divided across the days of the week may be less significant for children's outcomes than the sensitivity and responsiveness of fathers during their time together (7). Unfortunately, one of the most significant challenges facing America today is the lack of fathers in the lives of their children.

I never really knew my father growing up. I recall growing up in a nice house. I remember my father working and coming home. I remember sitting on the porch and watching my father come home from work. I remember standing in the door and watch my father wash the cars. I don't recall ever really having a father and son moment. It was something I wanted growing up, but I don't recall the special moment. If I had to describe my relationship with my father growing up, I couldn't. I don't recall my father ever coming to school when we were living as a family. I would see other parents together, but my father wasn't seen. It was a painful feeling growing up wanting a relationship with your father but never really able to develop one. Everyone in my neighborhood lived with both parents. We all played with each other daily. I remember those days. My father never taught me how to fight but he would fight my mother. I remember liking this girl in third grade. Her name was Kimberly Winfield. I would sit in lunch and watch her. She was funny and cool. I wanted a girlfriend. I wanted Kimberly. I wrote her a letter. I wanted to be her boyfriend. She said no! I was hurt. I stopped going to lunch. All my friends knew how much I liked Kim. She showed everyone the letter. I was ashamed. I wish my father would have been around more to help me. I remember one night my father whipped me for something stupid. He really put a whipping on me. He would talk to me while beating me. I could see years of anger in his eyes. His abuse became normal to me. I grew up scared to say the wrong thing. It would lead to a whipping. I went through my childhood in terror. I never really knew what to expect from my father. I remember waking up and going into the kitchen to get breakfast. My father was sitting in the family room happily eating pancakes and bacon. My sister was sitting right beside him! I was still mad. I was going to get my father back for those whippings. My father was eating and happy. I walked past and farted right on his food. I turned around like it slipped out. He was mad. I told him I was going to the bathroom. He got up and dumped his plate and I laughed all the way to the bathroom. My mother thought it was funny. I remember being picked on by this boy up the street. He would beat me up every day after school. I told my father, but he never did anything about it. It really bothered me growing up. It was like I didn't have a father in the house. My father was mean. I would get beatings for the smallest thing. He didn't waste time pulling out the belt. I never saw him give my sister a beating, but he tore me up. I do recall this one particular week. I remember hanging out with my friends around the street. We were smoking cigarettes. I was choking trying to smoke cigarettes. I decided I would take some cigarettes home and practice. I knew my father didn't get home until 5:00 p.m. so I was good. I was in the basement. I pulled out the cigarette, lit it up and began to walk up the steps. I looked up and there was my father. I almost swallowed the cigarettes. I finally thought my father cared for me. He didn't want me smoking. He said it would kill me. My father beat another hole in me the same day. I don't smoke today.

Finally, my father showed how much he cared. Any sense of caring from my father was good news to me. We continued to live in the nice house. The relationship between my parents was reckless, my relationship with my father wasn't any better. My mother couldn't do too much because he would snap for the least little thing. I felt like my father would take out his anger on me because I was close to my mother. I was mama's boy and my sister was daddy's girl. My mother never showed a difference in how she felt about my sister and me. This was mind-blowing growing up. I thought parents loved their children equally. I never stopped trying to be a good son to my father, but he didn't seem to care. I wanted my father to be proud of me. We continued to live in our house and my father produced another son outside his marriage. My mother was hurt. I was shocked. I wanted to see how much time he would spend with my brother. My stepbrother's name was Bobby. My brother eventually received the same treatment. However, because my father wasn't present, he was abused. My father was upset because his son was gay. He stopped communication with him. My brother's nickname was "Skip" and mine was "Flip." My father never brought his name up in a conversation. He was ashamed. My father didn't have anything to do with my brother, he basically disowned my brother. The cycle continued like water flowing down the stream. My brother ended up suffering from depression. He doesn't leave his house and can't function in public.

Meanwhile, I knew the marriage was over. My mother didn't leave, and I couldn't believe it. Finally, my father lost his mind. He was upset with my mother. He picked up the phone threw it and knocked her eye out of place. She was rushed to hospital. A couple of days later my mother left. I knew for fact I wouldn't see my father for a while. We moved right up the street to an apartment. We stayed one year. My mother became sick. My parents finally divorced. My sister decided to live with my father, and I went with my mother. We moved about 20 minutes away. My mother died four years later. I ended up living with my grandmother. My father very seldom picked up the phone to contact me. We eventually spoke on the phone. I wanted to see my father. I was excited. My father told me he was going to pick me up on Friday. I would pack my clothes on Thursday. He promised me for two years. I don't recall him ever picking me up more than 5 times. I would sit on the porch and wait for him. I remember seeing his car. I couldn't believe it. He pulled up. He said, "Junior, an emergency came up." He apologized and drove off. I was tired and hurt. I still kept the faith. I spoke to him on Thursday night.

I will never forget this conversation. He promised he would be there on Friday. I waited and waited. He never showed up. My grandmother didn't say anything. I've lost my mother. I didn't have my father. He would eventually come by the house to bring me money. I wanted his *presence* not his *presents*. I took what I could get from him. Our relationship was over the phone. I very seldom saw my father for months at a time. He never came to any of my school events. He never came to any meetings. He didn't know any of my teachers. He didn't even know my grades. I'm fourteen years and hurting. I went to school every day. You couldn't tell I was in pain. I was happy in school. This was one place I could go and forget about my problems. I was very popular in school. I was the manager of the football, basketball, and baseball team. The coaches became my stepfathers. The players became my brothers. I earned the name "Flip" while riding on the bus from a football game. We were always cracking jokes when we won the game.

I recall coming back from a win and I was joking on this particular payer. I was flowing and the whole bus was laughing. One of the players yelled, "You're crazy like Flip Wilson." I'm going to call you Flip. My father never knew how I became Flip! It's certain moments in a child's life where the lack of a father hurts more! My days were long. My days were sad. My days were like night and day. I maintained my hope in my father. However, other days I really didn't care what happened. I was losing hope! I would go in my room and cry thinking about what I did wrong. His problem was my fault. I graduated from high school. I don't recall my father coming to my graduation. I was a grown emotionally incarcerated young man. I decided to attend Charleston Job Corps in Charleston, West

Virginia. I wanted to get away! I was doing very well in Job Corps. My father would send me money every blue moon. He was cheap. He would send me five dollars and ten dollars. I begged to get the money. I couldn't understand why he was so cheap. He made good money.

His issue was all his women. I remember I called home. I needed some money. He told me I'm going to send you ten dollars on Friday. The money came in the mail. It was a 100.00 money order. I called my father so excited. I said, "Thanks dad, I really appreciate it." He said, "You deserved it, I'm proud of you." I spoke to my sister a couple weeks later. We were talking on the phone. She asked me about the money. She said the lady at the post office made a mistake on the money order. She added another zero to the money order. My father decided to keep the money order and send it to me. I didn't know what to think. Was he lying or stretching the truth? My sister was in college during this time period. She eventually graduated from Norfolk State University. My father was happy. He was a proud father. His baby girl graduated. I'm still tripping because he didn't say anything about the money order. I don't know why I would expect more from him. Regardless, he was still my father. I know he lied in the past, but I wanted to give him the benefit of the doubt. I ended up graduating from West Virginia State University. I transferred to Virginia State University and completed my Master's degree. My father was finally proud of me. We were in the kitchen talking one day I will never forget what came out his mouth. "I'm proud of you son, I've never thought you would do better than your sister." I'm thinking to myself this man is crazy. I believed in my father. I was a split image of my mother. The compassion, love, peace, and understanding for my father would never end. Our relationship became stronger over time. My grandmother who raised me passed. I purchased the house from all the family members. The city wanted the property. I refused to allow the city to purchase the house. I had to deal with the city. "Sir, you know it's going to cost over 50,000 dollars to remodel the house. The taxes are past due. How soon can you pay the taxes?" I handled my business the same day. I spoke to my father. I'm thinking about fixing grandma house up. He was very supportive. I told him what occurred when dealing with the city. He just smiled.

I was living in Maryland. I'm working on my Doctoral degree, working full time, and speaking. My father was instrumental in helping complete the project. He handled the money. He would drive down and check on the house. He made sure everybody was in place. He was finally my father. We were riding in the truck one day leaving the house. My father stated, "I made some mistakes growing up and I hope you understand? I wish I would had done things different." He never said he was sorry. I was glad he saw the error of his ways. I ended up totally rehabbing the house. I remember my father walking through the house. He would tell me stories of how my grandmother (Ms. Edith) took him in when he got out the Army. He told me if it weren't for Ms. Edith, he would have never made it in life. I could see the transformation. He was finally sharing. He was finally showing his emotion. He was my father. It took me six years to complete my Doctoral degree. My father told all his friends, "My son is going to be a doctor." He would brag to everybody. My father came to my graduation. He took pictures. He took extra copies of the program.

Our relationship was better than ever, finally. I decided I wanted to write a book. I wanted to help other young men overcome the various obstacles and challenges in life. My father was very supportive. I wrote my first book. The book was titled *Post Traumatic School Disorder "Empowerment Strategies for African American Males."* I gave my father a copy. He started reading the book. He became highly upset. He stopped talking to me. His pride was shaken. He told the world about his son becoming a doctor. However, he never told the world about his role of not being a father. I told the secret. I shared the dirty laundry. I didn't share all of it, but enough. My father was mad. He stopped talking to me. I went back to my childhood. My father was repeating the same cycle all over again. He stopped being my father. My sister called and said I needed to call my father. "If he is upset because I told the truth the…….! I meant every word I said" and hung up the phone. My father and I didn't talk for months. I put the situation in the Most High's hands. I was done with him. It was the first week in December and my phone rang. It was my father. I was shocked because he wanted five copies of the book. He even wanted to pay for the books. I didn't ask any questions. A couple weeks later, I gave my father the books. My father and I were sitting on the back porch talking about the Bible, life, and being thankful. My father started going to church and reading the bible more. He loved Dr. Fred Price. He would send money to the ministry all the time.

This particular night, we talked about his childhood. His father wasn't in his life growing up. He never really knew his father. You could see the pain in his eyes. His mother was very promiscuous, and it bothered him deep down inside. My father also spoke about how proud my mother would be of me if she were alive. He kept up with my mother's age. I'm glad my father was able to release. My father wasn't going to leave this earth *Emotionally Incarcerated.* It's beautiful to watch men tap into their innermost self to heal. My father told me he wasn't feeling well. I told him to make an appointment to see the doctor. He continued having health issues, but he hated going to the doctor. He shared with me he was still having health issues, but I knew he would be fine. I remember seeing my father for the last time. He didn't look the same. He barely could walk and didn't seem like himself. I told my sister to keep me posted on his health. My sister would call me to keep me posted. I remember driving back to Maryland and

thinking how he was looking. I was happy my father and I
relationship was better. My sister called me worried about
my father. He wouldn't go to the doctor and his health was
getting worse. We talked on the phone and he promised me
he would go to the doctor again on Monday. My sister
called me, and stated Dad was in the hospital. My father
never made it to Monday. He died a couple of days later. I
couldn't believe it. We were just talking on the phone three
days earlier. After his death, I started self-reflecting on our
relationship. Our conversations before he died help me to
understand him better. I was thankful. My father wanted a
small funeral. My stepbrother didn't attend the funeral. He
was buried with his Dallas Cowboys paraphernalia. He
loved the Cowboys and so do I. I'm glad and I had the
opportunity to *"Dance with My Father"* before he died.
The whole ideal of **Man down Father Gone** hit home!
He was gone.

"Map to Mental Wellness Success"

The solution to fatherlessness, morality, immorality, and
broken families is compassion, truthfulness, love, faith,
commitment, and a relationship with the God. In closing,
my father spent his life hiding from his fatherless
childhood. In addition, I realized my father needed time to
heal from his childhood trauma. Finally, as I grew in my
relationship with God my father took notice. I'm proud to
say men who open themselves up to God will find healing,
hope, and life filled with purpose. My challenge to you
write the names of five people you trust. Consequently,
select two people out of the five. Furthermore, I want you
to journal your pain and pray. Finally, find a group or men
who want to heal. The goal is **starting** the conversation. I
call it a "Constipated Conversation." You may decide to
select one person and start the road to releasing unfiltered
trauma. We all need one person you trust to release.
Overtime, the release will set you free. In closing transfer
your trauma with truth and transparency.

4. McAdoo, J.L. (1993). The roles of African American fathers: An ecological
.   perspective Families in Society, 74(1), 28-35.
5. Hofferth, S.M. (2003). Race/ethic differences in father involvement in two
Parent families Culture Context or Economy? Journal of Family Issues,
246-248.
6. All The Fatherless Generation (2018, May 20). Retrieved from
https://thefatherlessgeneration.wordpress.com/statistics/
7. Tamis-LeMonda, C.S., Rodriquez, V., Ahuja, P., Shannon, J.D., &
 Hannibal, B. (2002). Caregiver child affect, responsiveness and
                    and engagement scale (C-Cares). Unpublished Manuscript.

Biography

Dr. William "Flip" Clay is an internationally acclaimed award-winning counselor. Dr. Clay has been featured on the Steve Harvey Morning Show (96.3 WHUR). After meeting Dr. Clay, the first Hispanic Supreme Court Justice of the United States, Justice Sonia Sotomayor, recognized Dr. Clay as an extraordinary role model and leader. Dr. Clay is the author of *Post-Traumatic School Disorder* subtitled *Empowerment Strategies for African American Males*. In addition, Dr. Clay is the author of The Diary of an Emotionally Constipated Man. In 2012, The National Association of Black School Educators awarded Dr. Clay with the National Marcus Forster Distinguished Educator of the Year Award. Dr. Clay contributed to the *"Transforming the Educational Experience of Young Men of Color Journal Series."* Dr. Clay holds an undergraduate degree from West Virginia State University and a graduate degree from Virginia State University. Dr. Clay is also a graduate Argosy University the American School of Professional Psychology in Washington D.C.

Contact Dr. Clay at flip@RhymingtoRespect.com

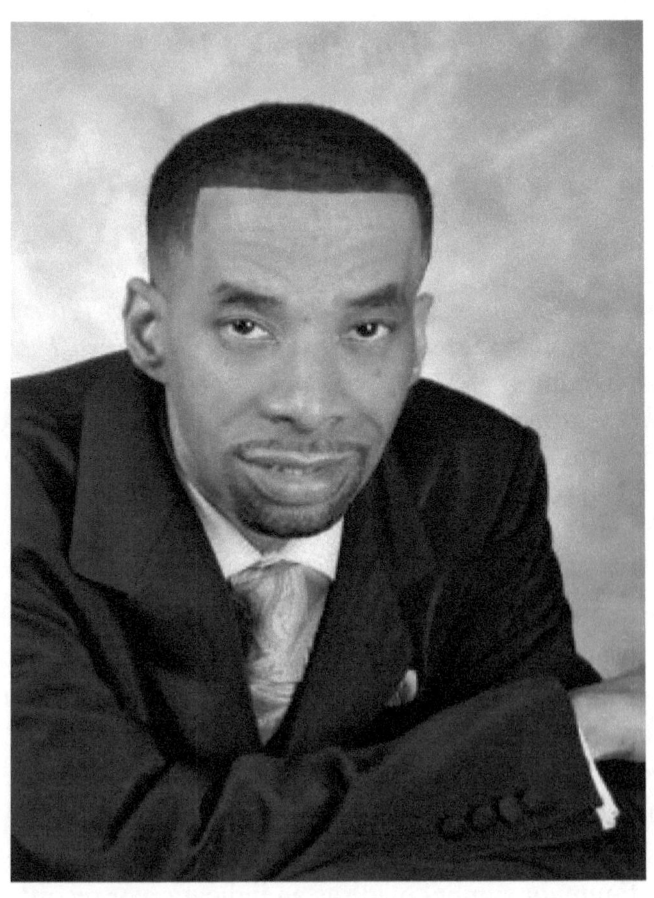

Chapter XIV

"The Mark"

Wendell Fields

Nickelodeon's Avatar: The Last Airbender (2005) Animation: Season 2, Episode 18 "The Guru/The Crossroads of Destiny" – Zuko's quote- "I used to think this scar marked me. The mark of the banished prince, cursed to chase... But lately, I have realized I am free to determine my own destiny, even if I'll never be free of my mark."

This quote says it all for me, Wendell Fields. This "mark" has cost me so many things. This mark has caused isolation, fear, anger, self-loathing, amongst many other issues. As I researched definitions for the word "mark", I discovered that it is defined as a small area on a surface having a different color from its surroundings, typically one caused by accident or damage. Another definition states a line, figure, or symbol made as an indication or record of something. When referred to as action verb, it states to make a visible impression or stain on. It is to write a word or symbol on (an object) typically for identification. These definitions come from the Oxford Dictionary. When I researched synonyms, I discovered these words: something is wrong, blemish, smear, smudge, dirty, blotch. Feelings and thoughts of being "less than" crept up or that something was wrong with me, I am different, or I am not like others. I am not normal became cemented in my soul.

Do these feelings and thoughts come to mind when you hear the word diagnosis? Or, what about when you hear the words, "You have this disease, illness, or health condition?" Honestly, I did not know what the word stigma meant; however, I discovered its' meaning by observing how people would treat others with a "diagnosis." I was associated with the outcasts… the "something is wrong with you, you are less than, I am superior than you, you don't fit in our circle" individuals. Being an individual bearing this "mark" of mental illness, i.e. depression, I experienced a battle of the mind, body, spirit, and soul. Because of this "mark", I have lost much, ranging from unaccomplished dreams and goals, a failed marriage, failed ministry, to some form of addiction i.e. food, sex, or even attention getting behaviors. I found myself attempting to take my life via getting hit by a train while driving. All of this because of my unresolved fear of being viewed as a "mark." But you know what, SO WHAT! As the quote says, "I have realized I am free to determine my own destiny, even if I'll never be free of my mark." In the words that emerge from reading this chapter of the book, you will discover how this 2 lbs. 10 oz baby boy would come to encourage, empower, and gain hope and freedom from the stigma, the naysayers…from those that would demonize, and those who would devalue a person with a disability or shortcoming of any kind. In this piece of writing, I share the story of the "chase." The chasing of several things that lead to self-destructive and self-defeating behaviors. Afterwards, I share some strategies and actions that I have taken to overcome the fear and *shame of self-stigmatization.* I learned how to use the negative energies and transform them into a positive voice, advocacy, and a symbol of courage and strength. I will be imparting 5 aspects that has helped me to form a foundation to stand on and grow by leaps and bounds. I hope that it will give a perspective that will aid in your growth to become the best person that you can be for today.

Do you remember Warner Bros American animated comedy series, Looney Tunes? Do you remember the elusive Roadrunner and the crafty Wild E. Coyote? I do too. It was hilarious! But that is how it felt with the "chase" I had been going through all the way up to my 40's. With me being afraid to acknowledge my mental health condition, to accept it, or seek out help for it, I felt like Wild E. Coyote chasing after the luscious Roadrunner of pleasure and acceptance. With being born 2 pounds and 10 ounces, I grew up small and skinny. I was always being commented on how small-famed I was. It bothered me and caused me to feel and think that I was rejected by others. I turned to food to cope. All it did was cause me to get fat and be talked about badly. With me feeling and thinking this way and not feeling good enough, the chase was on for the fast moving, smart, and oh so intangible feel for approval and favorable reception of another. It caused me to chase and to yearn for a feeling of wanting to feel better and one way was drinking. I was afraid to drink alcohol or use drugs. I had seen what behaviors came about from the different people in my life that chose to do such things. With there being a disposition in the family with alcohol, I knew that if I started, I would not want to stop. It was one of the socially accepted things that I could do and so I did. The drinking made the feelings and thoughts stronger and more intense. I could not control myself due to being under the influence of the alcohol. The feeling of not being good enough increased, not fitting in, and me considering myself as strange. After drinking one day, I remember becoming so sick to my stomach and my eyes hurt so badly. I remember all forms of light, rather electrical or natural caused my eyes to squint and hurt more. The loud noises caused me to feel nauseous and dizzy. It felt like the world would not stop swirling around me. I could smell the alcohol on my breath and coming out my skin. I decided

that I could not drink alcohol like that. I decided not to go
back to it or end up like family members i.e. dead. The
"chase" led me to pursue other pleasurable forms of
entertainment like sex. Oh, what I world it opened to me. I
become interested in having sex with women more and
more. The use of pornography came into play and it was
instant. Sort of like microwaved popcorn. I could get it
whenever I wanted it and as often as I wanted. I was trying
to deal with the ego driven hunger for my pain to stop. But
this led to more feelings of emptiness and caused
relationships not to be satisfying. I felt like I was only
good for one thing i.e. sex. I felt like the persons did not
like me for me and that their motive for liking me was to be
a notch on their belt, as well as, them being a notch on
mine. But it got old. With guilt and shame adding to the
list of negative feelings, it drove me to the church and to
work for my repentance. I became a Minister to fill some
of feelings of not being accepted. Although I was good
with ministering to others, I was not good at ministering to
myself. I still felt empty and ashamed inside even with the
victories that I had on the outside. I got married hoping
that it would stop the feelings of inadequacy. But it only
added to another level of "you should, you could have, you
ought to, you are no good." With these feelings continuing
in the marriage, my insecurities grew. I allowed myself to
be treated as though I was not a person but just a thing that
was to be used for whatever reason or purpose. I just
wanted to be loved and accepted. Can you say
"codependent." As I realized what I was doing, I tried to
gain back my individualism and fight back. This led to
arguments occurring more often. I felt like I could not get
any peace at my home. The thirteen-year relationship
ended in a divorce with a 3-year-old child out of it. My ex-
wife felt betrayed and her anger showed in many ways after
the divorce. I thought surely being a father and

concentrating on being a good father, would ease the pain. But after the divorce, an arrears statement was sent to me from the Services of Child Support. As I read it, tears started to flow out of my eyes from the statement saying that I owed child support and it was not true. I had to prove that I was innocent of such a thing. Thank God I kept the money order receipts that proved I was not lying. With being cleared of the wrongdoing, it left a terrible emotional and mental scar on me with the ex-wife lying on me. I started feeling less of a person and more of a thing. It appeared that I was good for something i.e. money. It was the only thing I could give. Everything I had put my hand to was crumbled into pieces. I lived near a railroad and started to have thoughts of ending my live with the use of it. My thought was, "At least you would be good for some life insurance money." I started to plan on how I would use the usual train schedule that ran throughout the week to my advantage to die. As the day came and I was committed to the act, the thought, "It will be over soon!" As the time came and I started to execute the plan, I remembered speeding up to meet the train at the intersection crossing. I wanted the train to hit me squarely so I would die instantly. As I got near to the crossing, I heard a voice outside of myself say, "Your son." It repeated itself loudly, "Your son!" From there, I can only remember turning the wheel and closing my eyes. The car turned and miraculously came to a stop. I found myself near a tree and a light pole. I was not hurt. The car had a dent but, appeared to be ok. I was shaking and I began to cry like a baby for an hour or so. All I could think was, "I need to get help!" I soon found myself going to a mental health facility to seek out help. There, I learned about "talk therapy" and how it could help me. But I found that it did not give me guidance for my life. It was a "whatever you like" type of feel. This type of counsel was not good for me, at that time. After

several sessions, I left. They tried to get me to take
medications and I refused due to fear of being stigmatized
and the side effects of the medication. I went for a few
years before taking another chance with medications. When
this time came, I was using a different insurance company.
As I was in the office and speaking to the psychiatrist, I
noticed a picture on the wall of two elephants going at it. I
asked why he had such a picture. He replied, what did I
see? I said I see two elephants fight against one another.
He said, "I see two struggles happening in one place. It is
affecting the area in which they are fighting one another.
The fighting was affecting the trees, grass, insects, and
other living things around them." The picture and his
words still make a difference in my life and reminds me of
how my mental health affects others around me with my
struggle. This helped me to decide to allow the use of
medication to help me. With taking psychotropic
medications for the first time in my life, I was afraid and
anxious. And it would prove to me that medication
compliance with this med, was a bad experience. It caused
me to feel "loopy." It was like the world was passing by
and I was moving so slow in it. I became afraid of man's
so-called technical wonders i.e. medications. This fear
drove me away from taking medications again. Time
passed. My job performance started to decrease, and
depression symptoms increased. My thoughts of wanting
to kill myself came up again. I decided to go hear a man
sharing his story, and his name was Kevin Hines. It caused
a desire for change to bubble in my soul. The job allowed
us to go to a mental health symposium where he was one of
the keynote speakers. He shared how he attempted to take
his life by jumping off the Golden State Bridge in
California. He expressed that while in mid-air, a fight of
emotional pain was at hand and how he wanted it to stop.
As he was in the air and falling, he came to himself and

said, "What am I doing, I don't want to die I want to live."
It spoke volumes to my heart, mind, and soul. With him
sharing how he had survived the fall and how he was able
to tell the story of recuperation, he sparked an
understanding and a yearning for a better life that was filled
with happiness, vision, and movement. After the speech, I
went up to him and expressed, "You just saved my life!"
He inquired about how but, I never told him. As he greeted
other people, I faded into the crowd like a thief in the night.
I thought I would never see him again. We would meet
again after a year or so of passing. He was doing a
documentary/film called Suicide: The Ripple Effect (2018).
It would show how he attempted suicide and the recovery
story that came along with it. He came to where I worked
to share the different types of community supports and
resources to aid people with managing mental health
symptoms, alcohol and drugs use, and developmental
disabilities services and the crisis intervention services.
When he saw me, he said, "I remember you" and I said, "I
remember you too." We hugged and I repeated what I told
him two years before, "You saved my life!" He responded
by saying, "But you never told me how." As I got ready to
share how, he immediately stopped me and said, "we are
going to put this in the film, and you are going to be a part
of it." At first, I hesitated and thoughts of people knowing
my business would come out. But I knew that change, is
not change, until you change. So, I agreed to share.
Afterwards, I shared that he saved me by showing that if
you attempted suicide and it did not work with ending your
life, what would you do. You would have to continue
living with life, just with other baggage that came along
with it. I explained that he gave me hope to change my
future and I realized that my destiny was my own to change
and control. He changed my thinking, perception, and
vision about life. Now with a change of heart and mind, I

can share with you 5 aspects that has changed my life and created a foundation to overcome the mountain of stigma, devaluing thoughts, feelings of rejection, doubts, and fears.

One aspect that has facilitated my success is the strategic use of prescribed medication. With the enforcement of film being shown across the world, it began to give me the courage to open my mouth to share with my supervisor about thoughts and feelings that I decided to give medications another try. Teresa Johnson shared with me how she was depressed after one of their parents had passed and shared the emotional turmoil she experienced. She educated me as to the name of her medication and expressed how it helped her to feel and think better with more clarity. I still feared the possible side effects that made me feel loopy as mentioned before. As I went in for the appointment, my "walls" were up; but I wanted to get better and I knew that I would have to face this challenge head on to get better. I was honest for the first time in a long time about my depressive thoughts and feelings and how that drove me to an attempt to kill myself. My doctor listened to every word I expressed. When doctor mentioned the word "medication", I shared my fears of taking such medicines without hesitation. I explained that I was concerned about the side effects, being labeled, and the different stigma that would come with my admission that I needed the medication in addition with admitting that I would acquire a diagnosis of depression.

The doctor glanced at me and gently expressed that he did not want to see me hurt anymore. He explained that my attempt to take my life was an indication that I wanted to do something about it. He expressed that he was there to help me, and we could take things slowly with dosage and the type of medication given. I remembered crying like a baby because I felt as if I had failed to manage the

depression on my own implying that I was not a real man…
a man who could manage his own problems. But as
Apostle Travis C Jennings of The Harvest Tabernacle
Church has said, "If you want something you've never had,
then you have got to do something you have never done!"

 At that point, what did I have to lose? I began taking the
medication. After about 2 weeks, I started to feel better. I
was able to concentrate on things better and not feel as
anxious or tired. When it comes to having a mental health
condition, I learned that the brain is either making too
much or too little of chemicals that help with managing
thoughts, emotions, and feelings, which can affect our
judgement and/or perception. I was now able to regulate
these thoughts, emotions, feelings, judgements, and
perceptions better in my life. After a month, I could feel
the difference. I gained the ability to express myself
without feeling "lost in the shuffle." Since then, I have
asked that my medication be increased, which has allowed
me the ability to function better with daily living skills and
abilities. It truly took great courage to admit that I needed
help and the willingness to give another shot at the use of
medications. However, soon enough I discovered the next
component to the puzzle of my mental health…SLEEP.

The second aspect of mental health is the component of
sleeping, not just the sake of getting sleep, but achieving
quality sleep. With having sleep apnea and being sleep
deprived, I learned that I was hurting myself and causing an
increase in mental health symptoms. I was not allowing my
body, mind, and soul to rest and replenish itself to some
form of normalcy. When I fell asleep, I would literally stop
breathing. Blood would not be oxygenated properly, and
this would affect physical, mental, and emotional
symptoms. As a way of getting air back into myself, my
body would wake itself up, causing me to toss and turn

throughout the night and not receive sufficient rest. With sleep deprivation occurring, along came moodiness, fatigue, irritability, depressed mood, difficulty learning new concepts, forgetfulness, inability to concentrate or a "fuzzy" head and more.

Consequently, I spoke with my doctor about the issue and he prescribed a sleeping pill but also insisted that I utilize a CPAP machine to assist me in getting the proper rest and quality of sleep that I needed to be healthy. I started to understand the purpose in being honest with the doctor and developing a rapport with him. But that brings me to another aspect to the puzzle of developing into a better version of myself. With my lack of proper sleep, physical effects began to occur. My eating habits started to emerge. As a result, when I was not resting, I was eating. The absence of an exercise routine, burning those calories, led to the development of obesity, heart issues, high blood pressure, and diabetes causing me to take a closer look at the perspective of my eating patterns.

The third aspect of the puzzle focused on my eating habits and consumption of types of foods that were not serving me to say the least. Of course, with there being a plethora of fast foods around me, choices for more advantageous and better-quality foods were scarce. When I mentioned the brain is either making too much or too little of a chemical, one's food intake has a lot to do with where we get some of the nutrients from. As the food pyramid suggests, eating more fruits and vegetables, grains, and less meat can help one's health and contribute to one's mental health. The choice of eating foods that are high in cholesterol does have a direct effect on depression and how that abnormal blood lipid levels can increase the risk of depression. High cholesterol can affect mental processing speeds, social skills development, the ability to be responsive instead of reactive, being able to self-regulate, and have self-awareness. That is why eating healthy is so important to my mental health.

So thus far, we have spoken about *medication compliance, sleeping, and resting, and the role of healthful eating* but, have we considered the pursuits and activities, that bring us meaning, purpose, creativity, and rejuvenation?

The fourth aspect that needed to be considered is the practices, rituals, and endeavors that bring happiness, fulfillment, significance, and value in our lives. I like to read, listen to inspirational recordings, look at inspirational stories, look at art, and be around people that add support and provide healthy value to my life. I enjoy drawing, photography, working out at the gym, and cooking a variety of meals. With completing and accomplishing these activities, they bring about skills, realization of what I can do, and helps me realize that I have the capability and capacity to improve my quality of life. These practices encourage me to not limit myself….to "really go for it" for lack of a better word. I recall seeing a dog that lost its front legs. I thought that it would be moping around and being inactive and depressed. But what I witnessed was a vibrant dog interacting with its owners and other dogs, playing with children, chasing after balls, and using its hind legs to propel itself into doing whatever it wanted to do. The dog appeared to accept that it did not have front legs. It's as if the dog said that its disability was not going to stop him from achieving a prosperous life. I looked at the dog and became inspired to acknowledge that I had a mental health condition; yet, I did not have to allow depression to victimize me into thinking that I was inferior, stupid, not worthy of, and able to act accordingly. I use one-word prints on tee shirts like Amazing, Influencer, Mogul, from my church and Kevin Hines tee shirts to motivate and encourage others at the job and wherever I go to foster hope. I had to learn not to focus on what I did not have and start to focus on what I did have, a brain that was capable of learning new things and applying them to my life and help others.

With practicing these types of endeavors mentioned, I have gained proficiency with different avenues which has resulted in building up my confidence, stamina, and willingness to participate more in life. I have gained meaning, purpose, and connection. Yet, there was still yet one more final aspect that has helped me to overcome the downward spiral of depression, and that would be learning how to utilize the natural supports of my community around me.

With the fear of being stigmatized and labeled, I refused to accept and acknowledge the help that was given in my community. Here it was that I worked in the mental health field for over 27 years. I heard and seen how coworkers treated individuals with disabilities. That fear limited me to remain in a small place of the mind. I learned that people are more apt to help you when you try and help yourself through confronting your own issues and being honest about them. I had to learn that I was not alone in fighting against the woes of a mental health condition. I attend various community supports i.e. mental health centers to see doctors, nurses, and therapists which help me to communicate about my physical, emotional, and mental health. I learned about the use of warm lines, crisis intervention numbers, local and national hotlines, and other additional supports. Rather it was online, through text, or phone call, that I discovered I was not alone. I participate in my local church to gain insight for my spirit and soul. There, I obtain purpose and gained meaning. There, I connected with others for a higher good and together, we get recharged and pour into the lives of others. I use the church, my job, speaking engagements, and volunteer opportunities in my community to assist in building connections, roads, and bridges to others that promote growth and expansion. Learning how to utilize my community effectively has caused me to grow into the full measure of the person that I am.

As we review this chapter, I've shared some fundamental concepts that have helped me to overcome *"the mark."* *A mark of negativity initiated by my fear, ignorance, pride, as well as the naysayers, those that would demonize me, or even devalue me due to my acknowledgement of a disability.* But guess what, "Lately I have realized that I am free to determine my own destiny, even if I'll never be free of the mark of others." Together, we noticed how medications can help. We learned how sleep and rest aids in managing mental symptoms. We discovered how healthful eating contributes to well-being. We saw how engaging in healthy recreational activities adds and funds growth in your whole being. Lastly, we observed how learning and using community supports supplies our growth to being the best person we can be. We are more than just one facet. Holistically, we are made up of different components which interact and thrive off one another. My hope is that you may discover what those inner and outer workings are so that the shine of greatness will cast its light to draw and save others from the turbulent seas of stigmatization and ruin.

I would like to thank my mother for being the first example of not allowing your mental illness to define who you are and what you can do. *My dad* for being able to say, "I'm sorry" when he was wrong. *My son* for helping me stay on this earth. I would like to thank *Kevin Hines and Teresa Johnson* for being examples of what courage is and the creative power of sharing your stories. *I would like to thank Viewpoint Health, Georgia's Crisis and Access Line* for helping with my growth and maturity. Also, I would *like to thank my sister, Cece Walker, Apostle Travis C. Jennings and the Harvest Tabernacle Church, C. Nicole Henderson, Mrs. Nadine Psareas and the Hopedealers Worldwide Crew* for supporting and encouraging me. I *would like to thank Mrs. Venessa Anderson-Abram and the platform of SDPPP Men and Mental Anthology,* for giving me this opportunity to share my thoughts, concerns, and ambitions to aid in paving a way of helping others obtain the freedom and love of life to be themselves and cultivate change from within out.

Map to Mental Wellness Success

There are different strategies that I used to aid me in obtaining my Mental Wellness. Here are some of the main ones I use. The approach that I use involves connecting with others. I connect with family members, friends, and organizations. My Pastor, Stephanie Jennings of The Harvest Tabernacle said, "Victory requires partnership." I must allow myself to trust others that add value to me and not debase me.

One way is through church attendance. In attending and participating in worship, I gain the strength and the courage to accept what the situation is. I listen to the Word as it is taught and preached; I connect the topic to different situations in my life. I take notes and review them. I search the scriptures for further understanding, guidance and for further ways to apply it. After this, I format a plan and execute it to the best of my ability. This helps me develop and cultivate my relationship with God. It helps me to be humble and to focus my energies on depending on God who is my Savior.

Another approach is having honest conversations with my doctor concerning everything. I do not lie to my doctor about my health. Although he will get on me about not following through with suggestions and advice, he is still there to get me on the right path of being healthy and being responsible for the farming of it. When the test result and lab results come, the truth will be told and shown to me so that I can make an informative decision about my health and how I want to proceed.

Another approach is *learning how to laugh. I have learned how to laugh at myself with making mistakes. I have learned how to laugh with people and not at people. I have learned how to surround myself with people who have a merry heart and who enjoy live.*

These approaches bring me to a place of wanting to further my search and involvement to use other avenues of gaining health. *It adds to my "repertoire and toolbox." Look out depression self-help groups! Look out Hotlines and Warmlines! Look out text lines! ONE STEP AT A TIME, I am coming for you! And, I will add you to my collection of helps!*

Biography

As an Engagement Specialist at Viewpoint Health and as a Field Care Consultant at Behavioral Health Link of the Georgia Crisis and Access Line, **Wendell Fields** is a part of Georgia's leading, responsive, and innovative teams providing mental health services to multiple counties. Wendell has given over 27 years of service to his community in this field. Wendell relates and communicates from live-in experience and personal perspective. He has been diagnosed with Depression and attempted suicide. Wendell understands the feelings, thoughts, and behaviors that may lead to one saying, "Forget this thing called life." Wendell has obtained a Certification as an Instructor in Question, Persuade, and Refer (QPR) Training which helps to educate and bring about awareness about the issues of suicide. Wendell has also been in the multi-award-winning documentary/film Suicide: The Ripple Effect (2018) with Kevin Hines. In the film, the collaboration brought mindfulness to the effects of suicide to the world. This film fosters a hope in storytelling as a way of creating a ripple of change, courage, strength, and so much more. The film has been played in theaters, schools, and colleges around the world and continues to cause impact. Wendell has been on various mental health panels, interviews on podcasts and radio shows, school events, and has been one of the main speakers at one of the Leadership Gwinnet's Main Event. May his inner buoyancy and compassionate flame, warm you, ignite you, and connect you to a purposeful life to share your genuineness, your warmth, and your passion with others.

*Renew your sense of confidence to overcome the stigma, naysayers, and those who devalue a person with a disability or beyond. I present to some and introduce to others, **Wendell Fields.*** Contact Wendell at wendell_fields@yahoo.com

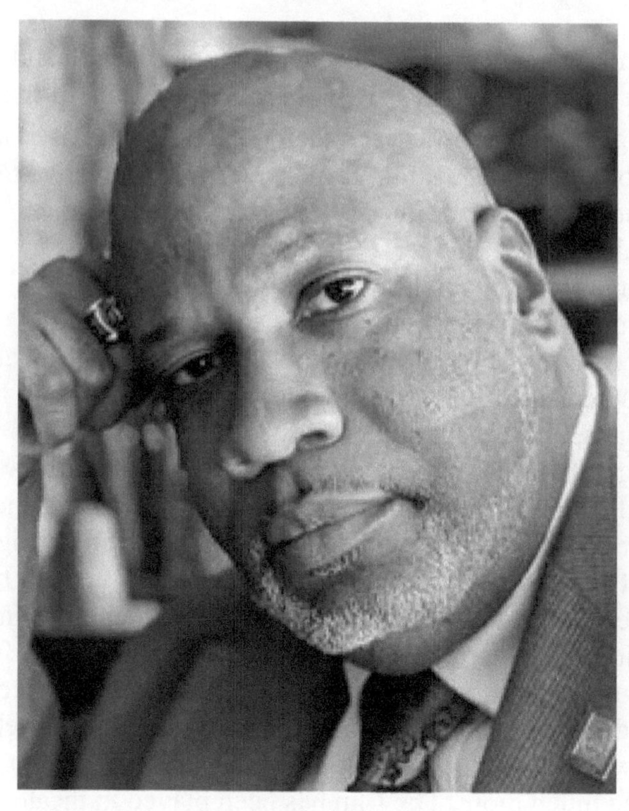

Chapter XV

~*A U T H O R S P O T L I G H T*~

Suffering in Silence

For God is working in you, giving you the desire and the power to do what pleases him. Philippians 2:13

Anthony L. Abram, Sr.

Hello, my name is Anthony Abram, Sr. One of my favorite things to do every day is go to the gym and workout. If I'm not working out, I love to spend time with my family eating at different restaurants and catching new releases that hit the theaters. There was a time when I did not understand mental illness until my wife was diagnosed. I realized after self-reflecting, I too, had been suffering in silence.

In 2018, I was off from work for a period of time due to my wrist surgery and noticed that I was not myself. I was easily irritated, angry, could not sleep some days and could not get out the bed many days. I became very depressed and full of anxiety. As I got closer to returning to work, I just became so overwhelmed about returning to the department I was in and fell deeper in a depressed state. I talked to my wife and she told me to contact the Behavioral Health Department and talk to someone, and I did just that. I was very hesitant at first, but I pressed through and found the nicest caseworker that was able to help me identify my pain, and this resulted in me being vulnerable, honest and transparent so I could go to the place of deep hurt and pain to start the healing process.

I was diagnosed with Post Traumatic Syndrome Distress, Major Depression Disorder and Anxiety. To be honest, I was not aware of any of these symptoms and became educated quickly. Depression is like carrying a one-hundred-pound sack on your neck, that's what it felt like for me! I always thought depression was for *weak* people and you had to be a certain way, but here I am…….

All of the above. I needed help ASAP!!

After speaking with my caseworker, the ball started to roll and I started to make appointments and see MED (Psychiatrists) Doctors to see if the medicine would have any effect on my diagnoses, and it did. I was scheduled to attend group session which I had no idea on what that would be like. I found myself incredibly happy to be able to see like-minded people, expressing their issues out loud and being transparent. I shared my story with my children and wife, and they were really supportive and encouraging.

I did notice that **advocating** for myself was especially important. For this reason, I asked a lot of questions and did my research on side effects of medicine being prescribed while talking to the doctor, as well as which facilities I selected instead of them telling me what they wanted me to do. I started the meds and felt they were not working, which it was suggested that I take the meds for about two weeks to start feeling the effects of the prescription. During this time period going to the gym was my only outlet.

Finishing the group therapy really gave me a different perspective about Depression, P.T.S.D. and Anxiety. Bottled-up feelings, on top of stress, and past hurt can really drive a person to become something that they could not recover from. That's why having a good support system while going through the tough days, really makes all the difference in the world. I have completed my mental health plan now I'm using my coping skills to remain positive while being conscious of things that will trigger any emotions relating to past experiences. That's why I choose NAMI and SDP3, these organizations focus on mental health, wellness, and peer recovery. Being active in those programs resulted in me learning how to share my story without shame, but with courage and resilience. I encourage you to learn about your mental health, for there is **No Health Without Mental Health. Men, we have a voice to stop the stigma and silence the shame connected to mental illness.**

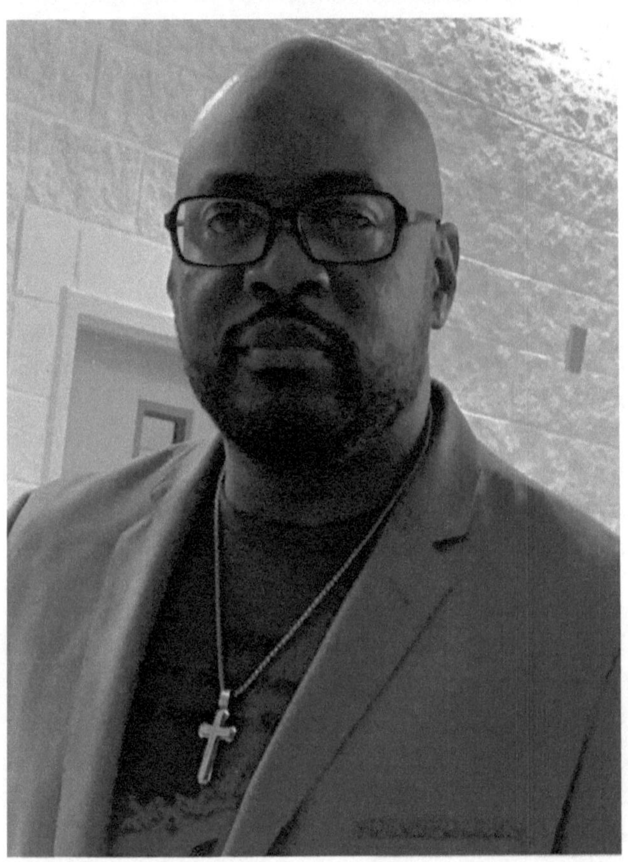

Chapter XVI.

And the Walls Came Tumbling Down

Bradley L. Candie

**Hope is seeing the light in spite of
being surrounded by darkness.**

It was storming outside as I made my way up the stairs to
my apartment…1136 Kennebec Street, Oxon Hill,
Maryland. It's funny how some things are clear and crisp in
my mind while others are distant memories. There are
certain sounds, images, people, thoughts, and feelings that
have never left me. All I have to do is close my eyes and
breathe in and I'm right back in my apartment. I can't
remember the exact apartment number though. I do
remember living on the second floor above Ross'
apartment. I guess that's a blessing to some degree. I have
fond memories that flood my mind of the times spent here,
but other memories I pray to God to erase forever. There
are certain experiences that I believe God allows me to hold
onto to as they can serve as a constant reminder of where
I've been and *how I got over…my soul looks back and
wonders how I got over.*

I will tell you this now that as I recall *And the Walls Came
Tumbling Down*, I will struggle to stay focused. I will
choose to talk about other intrusive thoughts and feelings
that impulsively entered my mind to protect my sanity and
to give my soul a break from the resurfacing pain. I have
the right to do that. I've learned to do that…to protect
myself from the trauma I lived through and *survived*. I will
protect myself from others and even me. This will not be an
easy task to undertake, but it is necessary. I pray it will save
lives as it did mine.

Now let's see, where was I? Oh yes, I struggled to make my way up the stairs to my apartment. I was hurting inside something bad but couldn't put my finger on *why* and *where*. The hurt was tangible. It felt like I could just reach inside and pull it out. Believe me, if I could, I would have. The thing is, I didn't know where the pain was. I knew it was there but couldn't pinpoint exactly where it was. Have you ever hurt so badly inside and wished you could clinch the pain in your fist and squeeze the life out it? You just wanted that pain to stop. You wanted the hurting to stop. Even if the pain wouldn't go away, you just wanted a break…temporary relief from the daily torment of unbearable, relentless torture. Everything was hurting…my mind…my heart…my entire being was riddled with an excruciating pain that was trying its best to destroy me from the inside out and was succeeding. As I made my way to my apartment door, I leaned against it for support with tears streaming down my face.

"God, please dear God…take this hurt away from me," I prayed like I never prayed before and perhaps it would be my last. "Please…if you care anything about me, please take the pain away."

I have to admit, my faith was wavering. I had been praying this prayer over and over again and it just seemed like God had forgotten my name. Was that even possible? After all, He named me. He called me. He gave life to me and He never answered. I must have waited for what felt like hours at my door, but in reality, it was only seconds…enough time to catch my breath and wipe the tears from my eyes so I could see how to unlock my door and press on. I can still hear that eerie, squeaking sound of the door opening followed by a chilling breeze brushing past my face reminding me that I was alone. Within the hollowed walls of my apartment, I was met with darkness. That same darkness that lurked in my heart. I shut the door, locked it, and prayed one more time.

"God, can you hear me? It's me, Brad. I need you Lord right now. I can't wait another minute…not even a second. My life depends on it!"

I know…I know, you aren't supposed to talk to God like this and never are supposed to demand anything from God…or at least that's what I was taught growing up, but when you get to the point of desperation like I was that night, and I hope you never will, you will say and do anything to stop the pain. Honestly, if I could have made a deal with the Devil himself, I would have. *Don't judge me!* Get to the point of giving up…wanting to die and talk to me then. Yes, me, Bradley Candie, …a Morehouse Man, Graduate of Howard University, grew up and served in the church, brother of Alpha Phi Alpha Fraternity, Incorporated, son of Fred and Gertrude Cox, Deacon, Minister, and on and on and on…*I WANTED to DIE!*

Now that I have your attention, here's the disclaimer. I am sharing my personal life with you. I ask that you respect me, and all the information found within these pages. Yes this will be a prime opportunity for you to gossip, say *I told you so*, judge and even lie on me, but all I ask kindly from you is to give me the dignity I deserve in sharing my journey to wellness and if by chance you read something that provides comfort to you, gives voice to your internal suffering, sheds some light on the possible struggle you have seen someone else go through or simply begins a conversation with someone else attempting to answer the question *why*, you handle my journey and the journey of others with compassion as well as keep the dialogue going. You see, there will be those of you who will read this story and find the mirror reflecting back at you. You will be able to sympathize with me. You will have walked in my shoes and you perhaps will feel that I am telling your sworn confidential thoughts and feelings behind the mask of happiness you wear on a daily basis to play like everything is alright and your life is great and free from worry. *If that* *is your truth, **remove the mask** and take the steps necessary to heal.*

The door shut sealing me in my apartment…my supposed to be early coffin. I was alone and I couldn't stand the person sharing the silence with me. It's a shame to say it, but I couldn't stand being alone with myself. I was worn down and couldn't take another step. I made my way to my black leather couch and fell into it like falling into the arms of a love one; however, there was no love being shone back. My bags from the day still clung to my shoulders weighing me down like cement bricks pulling me to the bottom of the ocean with no one caring that I was gone or even noticing I was missing. My clothes were saturated from the storm outside. My breathing was labored. My heart was raising. I was dying. It was a slow, painful death. The kind of death that lingered around like buzzards awaiting its prey to surrender and take its last breath.

"God take me now." I whispered into the fold of the couch.

I made up my mind that there was no coming back from this bout of depression. I had faced and fought this demon many times before and was victorious…or at least I thought. I just didn't have the energy nor the will to fight again.

"God, please. I'm so tired."

I can remember crying to myself because God sure as hell wasn't with me. Everything that I had been taught as a child concerning God, God's Mercy…*He may not come when you want Him, but He's always right on time*, was a crock of *SHIT* to me! Yes, I said it and meant it at the time…or at least I thought. I was wishing for my death and the *One* that I was told could save me and set me free was nowhere to be found. Was He just sitting in silence feeling sorry for me? Was He laughing at my pleas and found my suffering amusing? Was He really reaching out to help me in my time of need and I just didn't see His hand?

127

"The hell with you God!" I remembered screaming from the top of my lungs, but still looking around the room for some sign…a signal that He was near…that He was with me.

The silence was brutal. I couldn't shut out the echoing of failure in my head and the thoughts of not being good enough. No God. No relief. No change. Just relentless pain and unyielding sadness that gripped my heart and wouldn't let go. I remember sitting up and staring out the sliding glass door. It was pitch black outside. The only light that somehow parted the dark abyss was the lighting that lit the sky as the storm seem to subside. Funny, the storm outside was dying down, but the storm in my heart raged on.

"Well, if you're not going to speak to me, I'm gonna-"

I couldn't say *it* out loud. I have thought of *it*. I wished for *it*. I even dreamed of *it*, but I just couldn't get myself to say,

"I'm going to kill myself."

Was I really at that point? This was *it*. You have to be careful of what you put out in the atmosphere. Once the fatal words parted my lips, it released a flood of thoughts that I never experienced before. Immediately, I started thinking about *how*. You see, I never got to this point. The point of actually acting on the intense, impulsive thought of killing myself. I became consumed by *it*. It was like the damn holding back tones of powerful, raging water yearning to be free had broken and began flooding every crevice of my mind. I was focused and fixated on the thought of killing myself. It was intoxicating and enticing. It was a rush. It was exhilarating. It was…the end? Was I actually going to do it? Was this about attention? Was this real? What was I thinking? When? How? Will it hurt? Will I feel anything? Will it be fast or slow? Did I have the guts? Will they miss me? Would anyone care? Who would come to my funeral? What would they say? Will my family understand, or will they be angry with me? I was suffocating…hyperventilating. I stood up with such determination that it startled me. I wasn't in control. The quest for the *how* drove me insane.

"Calm down," I said to myself. "Breathe…Breathe!"

I remember walking to the balcony window, opened the sliding glass door and walking outside. It was dark…so dark outside. The thought of maybe jumping from the second floor entered my mind.

"You're not going to do that Brad," I convinced myself. "Do you really think that you would jump?"

I was talking to myself…carrying on a conversation with someone that was irrational and not thinking clearly but was most definitely in control. I had to appease the irrational me and comfort the hurting me and make a decision that both would agree to. I ran back inside slamming the sliding glass door behind me and stood in the middle of the living room panicking. The thought was still there, but the *how* still wasn't clear. Pacing back and forth from the couch to the table to the kitchen back to the couch almost drove me crazy.

"I'll shoot myself!"

I stopped in the middle of my tracks and seriously considered shooting myself.

"Brad, you don't have a gun."

By this time, I was exhausted and collapsed back into the couch…bags still clinging to my shoulders and I was sinking further and further down. I closed my eyes hoping…praying to hear God's voice in the stillness of the night. I couldn't even commit to whether or not I wanted to believe in God or turn my back on God.

"Where are you?" I screamed one more time.

Hope…hope is all that I had to keep me going day in and day out. When a man…or woman, boy or girl…when a person no longer has hope, there is nothing keeping them alive. God, for me, was the hope on which everything was built. No, it was not fair for me to place so much on God and so little responsibility on myself, but that lesson came later…much later in life. The only thing left to do now was to go through my *valley experience* alone.

This was my last attempt to hold onto my faith because what came afterwards, came with such force, such resolve, such determination that it convinced this weary soul that the conceived plan implanted in my spirit was *it*…my freedom from all the pain. Everything seemed to move in slow motion. Even the storm raging outside my window appeared to yield from its thrashing against my windowpane. This realization of the *how* seemed to calm by internal turmoil. Ironically, there was this sense of peace. The phone didn't ring. No one knocked on the door. There was no intervening from God to let me know that this was not my purpose or His plan for me. What was clear was the *how*.

I dropped my bags at my feet, wiped the tears from my eyes, looked around as if trying to take in what was going to be my last memories of my life and walked to the bathroom. I stood in the doorway, flicked on the lights, and glanced at the man staring back at me in the mirror. I didn't recognize him at first. Blinking several times cleared my confusion. That man was me. I could see the young, bright-eyed boy who was filled with so much life and passion slowly fade into the background. What replaced him was horrifying. Who was this withered, unkempt shell glaring through the cracks in the mirror? I shook my head attempting to jar the image from my mind, but as I shook more violently, so did he. I hunched over in on last effort to give God a chance to save me from my set-out plan. By this time, there was no screaming. I didn't have the energy for it. I was tired…so very tired.

"If you care about me God, stop me."

I was by myself. *I was afraid that I was going to be successful knowing that I didn't really want to die. All I wanted was to release this heaviness.* I was so, so burdened down. I couldn't bare the weight anymore. I couldn't breathe anymore. With my last once of strength, I faced the man in the mirror and smiled.

"You've won."

He laughed back and said,

"I know."

I slowly opened the cabinet revealing a bottle of pills. What kind? I'm not even sure. It doesn't even matter. I embraced the bottle, took the cap off, held it up to God and-

My name is Bradley Candie and in 1996, I entertained the thought of suicide and to my recollection, made the attempt. I say made the attempt, but I am not entirely sure if that is accurate. You, see, I did walk into my bathroom, found a bottle of pills, removed the cap to the pills, held the bottle up to God and from there, what came next was more than a blur. I have no memories after that. What happened next was not for my eyes to see. When I woke, I discovered that it was the next day and I was laying in my bed unharmed. How could this be? I was alive. I couldn't explain it. I was *alive*. I have chosen to believe that at some point in time, God intervened on my behalf. I genuinely believed that God had heard my cries and knew that I was about to yield to the overwhelming pressure in my life and was resolved to killing myself. I have chosen to believe that God waived his mighty hand over my eyes shielding me from the war raging around me and within me. Thank God I wasn't successful. It took me years to figure out that although I had a plan, God had a *purpose*. His purpose for me was greater than the pain, however, I had to go through the process to get to the purpose…my purpose.

You see, I did not come from a traumatic background or a broken house. I wasn't beaten, molested, abused, or abandoned. My mother did not neglect me and allow the streets and whomever walked them to raise me. She did not permit man after man to come into our home attempting to discipline me by any means necessary. I didn't see my mother abused and mistreated by my father. My father was not incarcerated and absent from my life. I did not yearn for the presence of a male figure to replace the void of not knowing or having a father present. I was not orphaned and abandoned for the system to raise. I did not move from place to place with no sense of a foundation. I am not a product of alcoholism and/or drug abuse. I did not come from a dysfunctional home filled with chaos and confusion. I did not want for food and shelter and had to do anything to get it.

I came from a two-parent household and a loving and supportive family and community. The *Tribe* definitely raised this child. I wanted for nothing. I was encouraged to do the best that I could and was taught to be proud of myself. I was exposed to resources that assisted me in obtaining the best education afforded. I observed how a mother having to work cleaning up after people who would degrade and disrespect her, fueled her desire for a better life for her child. I observed how a father who worked hard every day of his life used his aches and pains to teach his son the value of hard work and the importance of a good education. I was shown that I was loved. I witnessed parents sacrificing for their child and benefitted from the lessons taught about showing compassion for others and being your brother's keeper. No, my life was not perfect and absent from family strife, but it was a *good life.*

The question remains, how did I get to the point of wanting to kill myself? Sometimes the contributing factors are not so overt and noticed by the naked eye. Was I predisposed to such a mentality or was it the old argument of *nurture verses nature*? The more I think about what contributed to that horrific night and what led up to the decision to act on the thought to kill myself, the more I realize that I never really *loved* and *valued* myself. I have always struggled with not feeling good enough. I have always paid more attention to the negative comments of others than I did to the uplifting and encouraging comments from family, friends and loved one. I always sought the approval of those who didn't care anything about me. Not only did I seek their approval, I allowed them to help shape my internal image, my worth and value. I was a people pleaser and a caretaker.

I would fixate on the negative comments heard. *He's ugly. He's to skinny. He has a big head. He's gay. He's not black enough. He's not hard enough. He's soft. He's that way. He thinks he's better than us. He thinks he's smarter than us. Why does he dress that way? He's funny acting. Why do you talk that way? Why do you act that way? He's a Nigger. He want's to be White like us. You can't be gay and serve the Lord. Be a man. Straighten up. Don't cross your legs like that. Men don't sit like that. Men don't stand like that. Do you like girls? I bet you like boys. Sissy! You're going to Hell.* As a child, I didn't know what to do with all of these questions, thoughts and feelings that were running around in my head. All I could do was keep them safely kept away behind the walls in my mind. I compartmentalized the different facets of my life and did my best to ensure that the worlds never met unless I wanted them to.

The driving force behind all my poor decisions in my childhood, adolescences and adulthood was my low self-esteem and worth. Words are powerful. In my head, I honestly thought and believed that I was this ugly person people talked about. My focus was on the exterior and not building what couldn't be seen. It didn't matter to me that I possessed positive attributes. I didn't fit the imagine of what society said I *should* look like…what a man looks like. I was extremely hard on myself. I didn't look like what others said was attractive. I never took the time to define what attractive was to me. This was and turned out to me dangerous.

Coupled with low self-esteem, I knew at an early age I was GAY. It was hard enough being a confused, black, male with low self-esteem trying to please and appease everyone. I was also gay. Times were different. Unlike today, people, or at least the people that I knew were gay, were not open and *out of the* closet. They hid it like a family secrete. With all that was going on, in my head, I quickly learned how to wear a mask. I tried to blend in, but it didn't work out well for me. This really didn't help my situation at all. You see, when you wear a mask for too long, you sometimes forget who you are underneath. You question who the real person behind the mask is. You morph into a conglomeration of fantasy and reality. Not only did I wear a mask, the mask changed depending on who I was around. Some days I fitted in as best I could and other days I didn't. The days fitting in and being accepted, or at least I thought, felt so good. I wasn't talked about and singled out. I wasn't laughed at. I never wanted to take off the mask and step back into my harsh world. Unfortunately for me, my fantasy world was short lived and most of the time I was forced back into my reality. Don't get me wrong, I had plenty of friends and people in my world that loved and supported me. Remember, my fixation was on the few people who teased me and didn't love me.

I tried talking to my family and friends, but it didn't help. Maybe it didn't help because they saw the beauty in me. They didn't see anything wrong with me and didn't want to see me hurting. They knew that this was a passing stage and that I would get over it or at least they hoped I would. Little did they know, I was disappearing right in front of them. I also realized that sometimes people are more comfortable with the idea or image they have of you then who you actually are. I tried to talk with my mother, family, and friends, but most of the time I heard, *You are so smart. You are not ugly. You have a bright future.* I always wondered if they were telling me the truth. I have experienced with my family them protecting me from the truth because they thought I would not be able to handle the it. They were protecting me from what? Didn't they know that I was already hurting and being attacked? Yes, they are supposed to say exactly what they said. This is how they were programmed and how they were taught themselves, but truthfully, I don't think they knew how to help me. No one talked about their pain inside. They just pushed it further and further down hoping that the bag would not burst. I call this the *generational curse.*

I learned over time that my immediate family, my mother primarily, couldn't really guide me because she was struggling herself. My mother always focused on the negative. She never appeared to enjoy life. She kept people at a distance. I never saw her hang out with friends. My mother would always say, *you can only trust a person a far as you can throw them.* I grew up with this kind of mentality. My mother had secret wishes…dreams that she kept to herself. I would often ask my mother what she wanted to be in life. She would smile and light up when she told me. Then the smile would slowly disappear when reality set in. She wanted to be a RN, but that aspiration never came true for her. Her defense was to say, *oh well, it didn't happen.*

My mother loved to sit outside and hated it when Winter came. Although, she was never diagnosed with depression, I believe she had Seasonal Depression. As long as she could be outside and not trapped in the house, her mood and disposition were better. She avoided talking about her overwhelming sadness. She avoided talking about how she hated the way people talked to her and about her. She would always say, *I know how to do a lot of things. I'm not stupid. I have feelings.* It killed me to see my mother suffering so much inside. She allowed me to see so many of her talents and abilities but would not share them with the world for fear of not being good enough and being laughed at. She too was a people pleaser. She suffered in silence like I did and didn't know how to let it out. What would have happened if my mother would have learned how to manage her sadness and didn't care…really care what people thought of her?

I say all this to say, how you are raised both directly and indirectly can and will shape the way you see yourself and the world around you, as well as how you maneuver through it. Two hurting people cannot heal each other. Two hurting people can hurt together and sympathize with each other but cannot heal each other. My mother could not help me heal because she was dealing with her own hurt silently.

What also contributed to me remaining silent was seeing how my family handled situations and people who did not fit the image of what they wanted for the person or that person to be. Although they would say, *we love you just as you are*, their actions said, *we love you just how you are as long as you fit the mold and plan we created for you*. There were so many contradictions. This is another reason for keeping the *walls* up and separating the different areas of my life. I heard how my family talked about gay people. I was afraid to seek guidance. I was afraid to voice that I was struggling with my sexuality. I knew how they would handle it. Although they would say the programmed response, *we love you regardless*, I knew their true feelings. I had to be…chose to be this perfect little boy. I couldn't add more to my plate. There was no more room. This wasn't just about being gay, it was about image…my family's and mine. I couldn't be this perfect boy who never got into trouble and always did things the right way and be gay. I learned to hide and define what was going on inside as *shame and guilt*. I learned to deny who I was. I learned to play the role of being perfect. I learned to suffer in silence. I learned to smile though the pain. I learned to assimilate into any situation I was in. I learned to be who others wanted me to be. I learned everything accept how to be me.

Here is the most painful part of the process; because I didn't know who I was, what I wanted and what I deserved, I entertained relationships that were unhealthy for me. I was never taught what a healthy relationship looked and felt like and how to go about seeking, obtaining, and maintaining a healthy, committed relationship. I believe it was assumed that being able to make good decisions academically and professionally equated to being able to make healthy decisions personally. Parents do not assume that your children understand what you are afraid or ill-equipped to teach. If you do not teach life's lessons at home, you run the risk of outside influences teaching your child the wrong information and this wrong information will be the foundation on which your children build their future. I did as such. I was never taught the *Birds and the Bees*. I was never taught that there is a difference between being in a relationship and just having sex with someone. My low self-esteem and feelings of low self-worth coupled with poor or no communication with my parents was a recipe for disaster. I sought out the wrong people. I had no healthy standards, morals, and values. I was not able to create and sustain any boundaries and limits in my relationships. I equated sex with love. I did not know my worth and allowed others to fill my head with meaningless, unfulfilled promises of intimacy and commitment. I placed myself in dangerous situation after situation seeking something and someone to fill the void in my heart. I was floating allowing the current to take me wherever and to whomever it desired to. It took me 50 years to realize that I could not enter a healthy relationship with someone else unless I learned how to enter a healthy relationship with myself. It is extremely difficult to unlearn unhealthy information while in the process of seeking a healthy relationship. I couldn't push pause or stop while I learned because life goes on. I tried not to seek the attention of others, but I was lonely with low self-esteem. I thank God for keeping me and helping me learn while in the trenches scared and wounded. It wasn't easy, but I survived to tell my story. **Please remember that just because you can't see someone's bruises doesn't mean that they are not there.**

What do you do when the very thing that you thought made you who and what you are is ripped right from underneath you? I was known for being smart, having a bright future and destined for greatness. I could always count on my talents and strong academic foundation. I could sing, act, counsel, run, and perform. I earned rewards, certificates, honors, and special recognitions my entire life. This was who I was. No one asked me what I wanted to do with my life. No one asked me if I was alright. No one asked me if I needed help. It was assumed that I was going to be more than alright. It was understood that I would select that path and equip myself with the skills and knowledge that would propel me into an amazing future.

I never thought that what had always been there my entire life would be taken away from me. I would be left with no core and no substance. After starting my post-graduate work in 1993 at Howard University, the truth of not really wanting to be in my program hit me head on. I knew when I graduated from Morehouse College that I had no desire to do post-graduate work. Honestly, I was afraid that I was not going to be accepted even though I graduated with honors. Once again, my low self-esteem affected my reasoning and rational thinking. I also realized that I did not attend Morehouse primarily for the education. I needed to break an unhealthy cycle that I was exposed to and lived all my life. I was trapped in my mother's negative thinking and depression and needed a way out. Academics was always the way. I needed to experience life and to have fun, but I was not equipped for life's planned pitfalls.

After starting my post-graduate program, I decided to leave the program because I didn't want to be there. This was the first major decision I made for myself. When I finally told my mother, she said, *I knew you didn't want to be there in the first place. I was just waiting for you to tell me.* This decision thrusted me into a world that I had never seen or experience before. A world that was to be created entirely by me. One would think that I would have been excited. Don't get me wrong, I was but my excitement was temporary. I found myself sinking into worlds that I had never imagined that I would be in. I did not have my academics to fall back on and to make me feel strong and powerful. This new territory was unfamiliar, and no one cared about me or my academics. The world that I thought I wanted to be a part of was not what it promised to be. I struggled financially, professionally, and personally. Once again, I was lost trying to regain my footing but never managed to.

You may be wondering how all this *stuff* is related to my desire to kill myself. During that fateful night where my life was changed forever, I did not have the ability to slow my thoughts down and reflect on all of my life's circumstances and dissect how each path taken, each decision made and each life lesson not learned played a part in constructing the foundation for that dark night. If only I had the ability to rewind the tape or even press stop before that night, my life may have played out differently. If only I would have seen the warning signs, maybe I wouldn't even be writing the chapter now. I am grateful for the ability to be able to recognize that I have an amazing life and had to go through what I went through in order to get to where I am and who I am today, however, I just wonder if some of the pain would have been lessened if only I was more aware and more prepared. There were many nights in which I sat in my silence and rewound the tape over and over again. I questioned what I missed, what I did not learn and what I ignored. In my silence, I became conscious of some of most critical factors that led me to a dark place where hope had dwindled away, and faith could no longer sustain me. Prior to wanting to kill myself, here are a few of the slowly simmering stressors that were present and ignored:

1. From birth, I was over protected. I was shielded from the dangers in life and never learned how to manage such dangers on my own.

2. Many of my decisions were made for me. I learned to second guess myself in ever decision I made in life. I sought the approval of others to validate me.

3. I saw that my mother was unhappy and wore a mask to protect her true feelings, but never learned how to step out from behind the mask and live life fully. Wearing a mask was the accepted way of coping.

4. I did not learn how to process the strong emotions that I was experiencing and was not taught that feeling emotions was appropriate, but what we do with the emotions tends to be the problem.

5. I pretended that everything was fine when it wasn't.

6. I did not talk about my feelings, but held them in.

7. When I attempted to share my thoughts and feelings, some people did not know how to help me, but would rather say *you'll be fine* .

8. I minimized the damage that having low self-esteem and worth had on my life.

9. Having low self-esteem and no direction made me seek validation and attention from others.

10. ***I was never told that it was ok for men to cry and that it was not a sign of weakness.***

11. I shamed myself for being me and not loving me exactly how I was created.

12. I did not allow myself to be an individual, but
always made the attempt to blend in.

13. I allowed fear to dictate what decisions I made in
my life.

14. I never developed a sense of self.

15. I knew my mother and father loved me but needed
to hear them say it rather than showing it.

16. I learned that love is shown and expressed by
buying things and not saying *I love you.*

17. I had experienced depression before and did not
know that I was depressed.

18. I did not know how to manage my depression
because I was told, *it will pass.*

19. My immediate family did not talk about their
feelings.

20. I always felt alone and sought the comfort of others
to fill the void.

21. I thought that sex and love were the same.

22. I filled the void in my heart with short term
temporary fixes.

23. I dressed up the outside and avoided dealing with
the problems on the inside.

24. I could not say no and mean it.

25. I did not set and maintain boundaries for myself.

26. I avoided dealing with myself and my problems.

27. I never learned how to engage in a healthy
relationship with a partner. I always selected the

person that I thought I deserved or represented what I was thinking on the inside.

28. I always trusted everyone even when they showed themselves to not be trustworthy.

29. I did not know how to stop placing myself in dangerous situations all for the sake of not being alone.

30. I did not have the courage to be me.

Each and every factor mentioned helped shape and mold me into that man looking back in my bathroom mirror. Can you imagine what it felt like holding in all that *stuff* and not knowing how to deal with it or manage it? I cannot change the past. Yes, I wish I was taught how to freely express myself without fear, retaliation, judgement or self-persecution, but I am thankful for the gift of life…my gift of life and the chance to pass on valuable lessons learned along the way. ***My purpose is to inspire and to not be silent. I have been silent for too long***. I encourage you to live life to the fullest and whatever obstacles are in your way preventing you from doing as such, have the courage and the wisdom to stay *move mountain. If no one has told you, you are worth the time and effort and have a gift and a purpose growing in you waiting for you to give birth. Your time is now.* Thank you for allowing me to share my pain and my joy with you. I hope that it has motivated and inspired to keep the conversation about mental health and wellness going. *We cannot afford to lose another loved one, friend, brother, or sister to the fatal clutches of suicide. I break the silence today.*
Blessings~

Map to Mental Wellness Success

Listed below are some of the key principals I have learned and applied in creating my inner peace and wellness:

1. Be true to who you are.
2. Listen to that small voice inside of you.
3. Find something or someone greater than you that instills and inspires hope.
4. Remember, emotions are not feminine or masculine. Emotions are a state of being and can be controlled by you.
5. It is ok to talk and to seek professional help.
6. Keeping silent is deadly.
7. Cry when you want to cry. Yell when you want to yell. Celebrate something every day that makes you happy.
8. Develop a strong sense of self and do not seek validation and attention from others.
9. Become aware of your warning signs and triggers and develop a healthy plan of action to combat them.
10. Boundaries and limits are important. Have them.
11. No man is an island by himself. Find a support system that loves you unconditionally and will be there for you.
12. Be careful of who and what you allow to be in your space. Words are powerful and can speak life or death.
13. Medication is beneficial for some and should be considered.
14. Celebrate your accomplishments.
15. Acknowledge your strengths and use them to develop your areas of weakness.
16. Meditation helps to bridge the gap between the internal and external.
17. Be active.
18. Don't be afraid to sit with yourself and listen.

19. Say I need help if you do.
20. You do not have to be everything for everyone.
21. Monitor your thoughts
22. Be kind and gentle to yourself
23. You are exactly where you are supposed to be to learn exactly what you are supposed to learn.
24. Remember, it is a process…your process. No one is going to do the work for you.
25. You were created for a purpose!

Develop your own map to mental health wellness. This is what I have discovered and practice daily. The best strategies are the strategies you develop and implement after your own personal self-discovery.

Biography

Bradley Candie is a graduate of Morehouse College and Howard University. Upon graduating, Bradley performed overseas in Mannheim, Germany. After returning to the states, Bradley pursued his passion for the arts and performed with the Atlanta Opera and theatres in the Atlanta Metro area. He has performed on such renowned stages as the Kennedy Center, the Philadelphia Academy of Music, and Carnegie Hall. Bradley is an actor, singer, model, minister, and playwright. His first piece written, *Sisters*, received recognition as a top five finalist in the Jubilee Theatre's 2012 New Works Festival and was accepted to be a part of the 2018 Las Vegas Black Film Festival. As a profession, Bradley is a Guardian Ad Litem with Fulton County Juvenile Court where he ensures that the voices of our youth are heard. You may follow Bradley on: Instagram @bradley.candie & Facebook @Bradley L. Candie

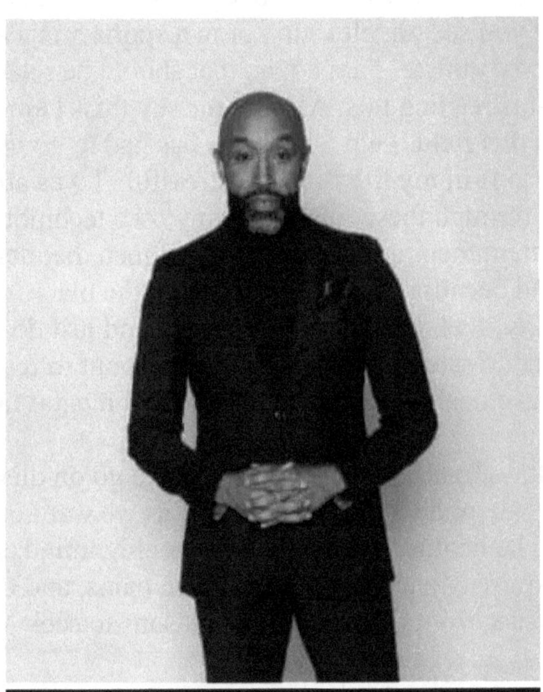

Chapter XVII.

Asking for Help is a sign of Strength, not a Weakness

James T. Thompson

Each Day is a Gift, the Gift is another opportunity to Be Better

My name is James T. Thompson. I am a husband, a father, a son, an uncle, a cousin, and a friend to many. I work 40 hours a week. I love sports, I smoke cigars and I like just kicking it with the guys. I say this to make sure that you as the reader understand that I am speaking as an average black man dealing with life as many of you are. This is not something coming from someone you see in a movie; someone you see on television or in a sports arena as a professional athlete. I am a man that should be relatable to most that is reading this. Also let me say this- I am not an expert in this field. I am a man that has had to go through some periods in my life that was stressful. I was able to navigate through these times with my own techniques of mental strengthening. I know of many men that deal with stress, and because of the stigma within the black community, feel they have to be strong and just deal without addressing it. So what you are about to read are ways I have dealt with, and even defeated mental fatigue.

The health of our bodies is the reason we go on diets, drink lots of water, and work out. Well just as we want our bodies to be healthy, we also need a healthy mind, and a healthy spirit. Mental overload, hidden pains, and deeply rooted issues from the past can be reasons to seek Mental Health.

When people hear mental health, they think depression, they think crazy, they think about being in a white padded room with a strait jacket. When people hear counseling, they think about laying on a couch and telling a stranger all of their business. That can be a little intimidating, might even be scary for some. I was that person. I was not going to sit on anyone's couch and tell them my business. When I speak of counseling, I try to ease the fear factor. I now tell people to open up to a dear friend, or family member. Doing this should help ease the fear of seeking professional counseling. Sometimes when you verbalize your thoughts, hearing them out loud can help. There are ways to self-evaluate and treat in these situations. However, counseling is the best way to treat these issues.

In regard to the mental overload, many of us black men will feel that is the normal way of life. We feel that we are the kings, we are the head of the household –all others are going thru it, so it is the normal way of life for us. We look at our fathers, our grandfathers and figure they suffered through it, so this is the norm. This is what we have seen, what we have heard –so we just deal with the overload. Issue is that without a release, the overload can reach a dangerous level. I have always heard that enough pressure will bust a pipe; well this is the same thing. In this case – the mental overload (pressure) will can create a mental break (pipe) and cause major issues. I've learned that as a man, and even more so as a black man, everyday life can bring stresses upon you that are not visible. The pressure to be a man -carry yourself as a man, protect as a man, provide as a man can be a heavy load to carry at times. Now as a black man –those same pressures *are doubled*. So Yes –this adds to that mental overload.

Let me give you a few examples
-looking at bills, wondering which one was going to get paid and which one would get paid next month.

*-is the bank looking for your car, or would they honor the
arrangements made for payment.*
*-wanting to ask a friend for a loan, but not wanting to give
the impression that you can't handle your business*
I could go on and on with regular life stuff that can be a
load on you mentally.

In my time, I was able to recognize this overload. Yes, I am
coming to you as a man that has experienced those things
plus much more. I was able to recognize that I needed to
slow down and create space within my mental capacity.
You may ask how were you able to do that?

First thing I did was pray and forgive myself for taking a
break from it all. You see, we get so entangled within
staying afloat, in surviving that we feel guilty if we are not
just trying to solve every issue at all times. Forgive
yourself. Then you should figure out something that you
love to do that can totally occupy your mind. You can look
for something new, but you do not have to. This can be
something you already enjoy doing. My things were
basketball, reading or watching a good movie. These things
took me away from the issues that were blinding me.
Afterwards, I was able to come back and view these same
issues with fresh eyes and a different spirit. I know this
seems too easy, but sometimes easy is what you need. Ever
heard of the saying –sometimes doing a whole lot of
nothing is actually you doing a lot of something? In this
case –chilling, relaxing, enjoying a hobby (which many
would say is nothing) is actually you are making mental
space (a lot of something) to deal with life. Now is this a
message coming to you from a professional –NO.
However, my method is free, and it will not hurt to try it.

Now the hidden issues from the past, is the one that usually
can't be self evaluated. You may ask why? The answer is
because you feel the issue is not there so how can it be self
evaluated. You see as humans we do not do well with

inflicting pain on ourselves. Example, you jam a finger and you usually ask someone else to pull it because all of a defensive mechanism built in that keeps us from inflicting pain on ourselves. Same with a hidden issue from the past. That issue was and is painful, so we bury it.

A few of my hidden issues:

- Growing up I saw the man in charge of my own home succumb too many pressures. I saw him lash out at the ones closest to him –me, my sister, and my mother.
- I did not have a mental disease; I had what I would call a mental situation. The absence of my father caused me to use most of my energies on doing the safe thing. I did not challenge myself enough to reach my full potential. Now did I do all things in a safe manner –no, as there were times that I did do the wrong thing. However, I always came back to a safe way of living.
- I lived with the motivation of not being a victim. Not being a victim of the no daddy syndrome. I refused to be a statistic, refused to let that be the excuse for a downfall. Again –at that time in my life, I was not a fan of counseling. So I self-counseled, and for the most part that worked.

I was able to be a good guy and grow into a good man. I became a father and did all I could to keep from being who my father was to me. The main thing I wanted to be was **present**. *I gave up career opportunities to stay near my son, I moved close to him so that I could be there when he called.*

Through all of this I felt I was happy. I am a man that loves being in a relationship. Yes, in my twenties…early thirties,

I had a great time as a single black man living in Atlanta. However –I always had fun with the goal of meeting that woman that could be my wife. In this time, I met many women. I mean –I met some great women. However, for some reason we did not make it. You would think that we did not make because of some big argument, infidelity, or something toxic. In truth, I am really unable to give reasons that these relationships did not work. I am sure there was a reason, but I am also sure that these reasons were something I made bigger than it was. In other words, I was sabotaging my own relationships. I was destroying my happiness subconsciously and did not even know it.

As I said, life was good. I was a good father, a good son, a good friend. My career was moving forward, making good money, I was traveling, I was enjoying life. Seemed I had all I needed. However, at this time I was still not able to fully enjoy life. I did not know what I was missing because I had never allowed it to be in my life. I was missing the ability to give complete love and also accept it.

This is where a higher power stepped into my life. It was a normal workday, but on this day I called in and told my supervisor I would be late. I was on my way in, listening to the radio. On this day, the guest on the show was a counselor that specialized in domestic violence and the children that survived domestic abusive homes. On my drive in, I stopped at a traffic signal not far from my work. A gentleman called in and said he was a child that witnessed violent acts between his parents. The counselor asked if he was calling in because he was abusive towards women. He said no, he was the exact opposite –and he could not stay in a relationship. This is why I say this was because of a higher power. I was not that far from my place of employment, and if I would have gone to work earlier in the day, I would not have heard this caller. It was as if I was supposed to be right where I was at that very moment. I felt that show was meant for me. That gentlemen calling in and saying he could not stay in a relationship weighed on me heavily. I thought about it all that day. The next day –I researched my insurance benefits and what mental health services were offered. I was able to make an appointment and see a counselor within the same week.

My first visit was almost stressful. I had all types of things going through my head -What am I doing? …Black Men do not do this….am I crazy…. How can this woman who does not know me help me…? will I have to lay on the couch? So, as you can tell –I was not a fan of counseling. However, that call on the radio kept replaying in my head. So, I just kept putting one foot in front of the other. This counselor just let me speak. She let me talk until I was talked out. One hour and a half, ninety minutes –fifty-four hundred seconds …words flowing. Afterwards she set me up for the next appointment. Now the second visit –we actually spoke. She helped me bring up the issue from my past. My issue was my father's absence. The very thing that I used as motivation to succeed and stay on the right path was the very same thing that was holding me back from complete emotional happiness. She did not tell me of the hidden pain, she let me discover it myself.

So, you may have guessed it, my hidden pain was not having my father in my life. It had been 34 years since I had seen him, and just recently I had started speaking to him. I made my mind up that I had to see him. With everything going so well, this seemed like the only thing missing in my life. I can't say that I needed a relationship with him, I did not need an apology –I just needed to either close a chapter or open up a new one.

So, I planned the trip –did not tell anyone about it, as I did not want anyone's opinion. However, I did tell my mother, sister, and girlfriend. I had to tell my mother, because I wanted to make sure that she knew this had nothing to do with her, or how she raised me. So off I went to New York to see the man that (in a twisted way) motivated me to be better and also was holding me back from being my best self.

The day I was set to go meet him was one of the most stressful days of my life. I had plans on going to see him and my relatives from that side of the family. Again, these are people I had not seen in over half of my life. I had no idea of how they were going to react to me, no idea of what they would say. No idea of how I would react -or how I would react to what they might say. I did make it through with prayer and the patience my God gave me during this day. There were things said that I did not agree with, there were things said that made me angry –however, through prayer I made it. I had no idea what this visit would do for me, no idea what was waiting for me on the other side.

Over the next few weeks and months I found out what was waiting for me on the other side. I can't really explain it, but I was able to see things with a little more clarity. I was able to love without limits. I was able to allow myself to be loved to the fullest. I accepted life without any regrets. This is what counseling did for me!!

There are many men, and even more black men that have lived through and is living through the same circumstances that I have. Many of us are living through it and not asking for help, because that is what we were taught, and what we have seen. We feel asking for help is seen as a weakness. Hear me…HEAR ME –asking for help is not a weakness, it is actually showing strength that not many have. Mental Disease is as any other disease, sickness out there. You have to recognize it, and then seek the treatment.

As I said earlier, I am not an expert, I am not a person with degrees on his wall. I am a man that has lived life and lived it through some circumstances that are more common than we know.

My name is James Tyrone Thompson, and I am a Man that believes in Mental Health!!!

Map to Mental Wellness Success

It is particularly important for me to enjoy life, but at the same time I like to inspire and serve others. I thoroughly enjoy the entertainment industry as a Host and Model. When I Host, I speak about the importance of mental health and seeking counseling. I am an Advocate of health and wellness and in support of therapy. As I model, this helps me plenty. Modeling is something I enjoy, and extremely passionate about as I walk the runway at my age. I believe I am encouraging others that anything is possible if only you believe. When I hit that runway -***I OWN it***. I feel as if I'm helping other men know you can do anything you put your mind to. I also read to expand my knowledge, watch a movie, or play basketball to get a physical release. Brothers, do know that there is ***"No Health without Mental Health", and there is no silence nor shame in seeking professional help.***

Biography

James T Thompson was born in Brooklyn, NY but calls Richlands, NC home. He is a HS graduate with 6 years of military service. After his military service he served as a Correctional Office in North Carolina. During this time he found out how much he enjoyed listening and sharing his experiences to help others.

James is a Model, a Host, an Actor and Author. Before all of that, he is a man, that lives by the motto -the Biggest Room in the world, is the Room for Improvement. He intends to improve each day in all aspects of life. Improving as a Father, Friend, Son, Brother, Relative...Man. With these improvements, He hope others can be motivated to be better themselves in that they do. He loves living life with a smile, as I feel we need more smiles in today's world.

James has a passion for helping out with younger men of and/or from single parent households, hoping to help them from a mental strengthening standpoint. Self worth is really important within our youth of today, especially of those from single parent households. James has been a volunteer coach at the Jr High school level, and helps with an organization called Future Gents -motivating youth through Style and Etiquette. He now Co Hosts a Podcast called Klassic Konversations speaking about issues within the community with hopes of solutions being sparked from the dialogue.

James can be booked by email –klassicjae@gmail.com
He can be followed on Instagram at klassic_jae and Facebook at James Thompson (Jae Tea)

Chapter XVIII.
The Fire in His Eyes

His eyes were as a flame of fire, and on his head were many crowns; and he had a name written, that no man knew, but he himself.
Revelations 19:12 KJV

Reginald Dale

On a hot summer day in Jefferson City, Mo, I was awakened by a series of nudges. "Daddy Daddy.. Dad…did you just hear what Cube said?" It was my 17-year-old son, Regie, Jr. He was looking me in my eyes with such a blank stare that made the hair on my arms stand up. He had been watching 106 & Park and was serious about Ice Cube speaking directly to him. I was trying to remain calm and keep my composure; thinking that any second, he would laugh, and say it was a joke. The laugh never came. It was not a joke, wasn't a prank—my son was delusional.

I took him outside so I could get his undivided attention and try to make sense out of what I was seeing and hearing. I asked my son if he was okay, but I already knew he wasn't. I called my mom in Illinois and told her Lil Regie was not acting like himself. My mom spoke with Lil Regie and agreed he didn't sound like himself and something was wrong. We planned to get him home to Springfield, IL because I was overwhelmed with all of this and needed the support of my family. To be honest, I was scared.

To get Regie Jr. on the Amtrak to Springfield was another can of worms of its own. He felt like everybody was against him. He felt like everybody was staring at him and intending to do him bodily harm. I had to hold his hand as we walked through the train station because if I didn't, he would wander off. And as I held his hand, tears were rolling down my face as I thought "Why my baby?"

After we arrived in Springfield, we took the ten-minute walk to St. John's ER. So, there we were, two grown men, walking down the street in the middle of the day holding hands. People were staring but I didn't care; I wanted answers. I wanted to see the fire in my son's eyes again. I had no idea of the journey that lied ahead of me. After some time at the hospital, the reality hit me; my son was indeed sick. However, it wasn't the sick we were familiar with. His physical body was fine; it was his mind that was ill. My son had a mental illness.

As I reflect to my childhood, I can vividly remember certain members of the community that were odd or different from the rest of us. I remember a man that I only knew as "Walking Robert". I am sure he got the name from the fact that he was always walking around town. Literally 24/7 he was walking. In fact, I can't remember ever seeing him stand still or sit down. Did he have a home? Did he have family? All these things flood my mind as I write this but as a younger kid, I never stopped long enough to answer these questions because it was someone else's problem not mine.

That is one of the problems of our society. We all have this disconnect when it comes to acknowledging, respecting, or just offering basic compassion to those with mental illness. There is a stigma. Why is that? Why is a person with a physical illness any better than those with a mental disability? Where is the empathy? Why is mental illness such a taboo subject, especially in the Black community? We treat our brothers and sisters with behavioral health issues as if they are second- or third-class citizens. They didn't ask to be ill; they didn't choose this life. It is just the cards they were dealt. I really feel that it comes down to a lack of education on the issue. We need more funding for research and to spread awareness, and more advocacy programs to reach and provide services to those in need. People are crying out for help, for adequate medical attention and therapeutic services. Just imagine being at war with yourself, in your own head. Imagine not being able to formulate or clearly and comprehensively convey your thoughts. I will be the first to say I was once ignorant to all the issues surrounding this and it took for this to happen to my son before my eyes were open to the injustices and prejudices we have as a society when it comes to mental illness.

It's as if we have grown to be casually familiar and passively accepting to what, without a doubt, has become the new norm. We all got that one person in the family that is "just not right". What about our socially awkward neighbor that is really nice, gives the warmest smiles but just doesn't seem to connect socially. Kids make fun and point out his awkwardness. This comes from a lack of awareness and a lack of education. I am sure we all have heard the phrase, "If you know better, you do better". So many times, I have prayed to God asking him to heal my son and let it be me that is tormented with the burden of trying to manage daily life with schizophrenia and bipolar disorder.

Back at the ER at St. John's Hospital in Springfield, I have just been introduced to a whole separate problem than the mental illness itself. My son has just been made aware that since he is 18 years of age, he doesn't have to allow me to admit him, so he's refuses treatment. Just when I thought it couldn't get any worse I had to convince my son that it would be in his best interest to let these strange people poke, prick, and pry into his world (his head) so we can make everything better. He wasn't going for it. I cried, hugged him, laughed, and cried some more. Finally, his mom showed up along with his other grandmother. They all tried to console Regie Jr. and trying to convince him to do the right thing. He showed no emotions, spoke no words. He sat there, half naked, in his reverse hospital robe, blankly staring through all of us. That fire that used to burn so brightly in his eyes was gone.

After what seemed like an eternity (7 hours), we were told that they would in fact be admitting him to the 10th floor. I was so elated because the last 24 hours had been so draining. I couldn't let him out of my sight so that meant no sleep for me because he didn't sleep. No one was allowed to stay overnight with him, so we showered him with some love; it wasn't reciprocated. Sleeping that night was even more difficult because I felt like I was letting him down because I wasn't at his side. The next afternoon I made it back to the hospital I learned they had actually got him to take a few doses of his medication, but he wasn't himself yet. He seemed to just want to sleep. I took that as a good sign because sleep wasn't something he wanted to do before. I visited my son every day at the same time— 1pm—right after lunch. On the fourth day, he was sitting at the desk in his room rather than just lying in the bed or gazing out of the window. In his hand was a Bible; he was so deep in reading that he didn't notice me enter the room. When he realized I was there, he jumped up and greeted me with a strong, warm hug! I held him for a few minutes as we both cried. I kept whispering to him everything was going to be all right. After we let each other go, he stepped back, and I could see the fire returning to his eyes. He had more life in his eyes. He was no longer looking passed me or through me, but he was looking directly at me. We sat and talked for hours until they told me visitation was over. With each day I saw the medicines were working for him and, in essence, bringing him back to life. After the seventh day, he had his sense of humor back and we actually had a few laughs about some of his exploits that he actually remembered. With each passing day he got better, and I was told he would be discharged on day 14. I was so happy, so elated to hear that my son would be coming home.

It has been 12 years and we have had our share of setbacks in the first two or three years. It is common for people on psych meds to start feeling better and think they don't need the meds anymore, so they stop taking them. Well, that is not how it works. The meds are your pass, your permission to a happy, healthy life. These days my son doesn't miss a dose. I don't have to monitor his meds as closely as I have had to in the past. He knows his meds are his connection to normalcy. We have learned over the past 12 years to accept these cards that were dealt to us. In most card games you have a partner, I am definitely his partner. Even though his hand isn't the best, I have all spades and I got his back!

Anything to keep the fire in his eyes!

Map to Mental Wellness Success

My faith, my family, and my support system has helped me to own and utilize my map to mental wellness success. I would encourage you to find something you love and pursue your passion with purpose and tenacity. We are what we think, and we are WORTH IT!!

There is No Health without Mental Health!

No Silence.

No Shame.

No Stigma.

No Suicide.

Biography

Reginald D. Dale, Sr. is a middle-aged single father of seven that has had his own personal battle with his mental health diagnosis. He is originally from Springfield, IL. He has worked as a community organizer and activist in the areas of reducing mass incarceration and bringing awareness to mental health disparities. He received his training through the Gamaiel Network (the same organization President Obama organized).   He also mentors disadvantaged and at-risk youth with his organization, CUJO (Communities United for Justice and Order). He is an avid Scrabble player and self-proclaimed chef extraordinaire/foodie. He just recently relocated to Atlanta, GA with his kids and his furry best friend, Boss, a 6-year-old Pug/Shih Tzu mix. He plans to pursue acting.

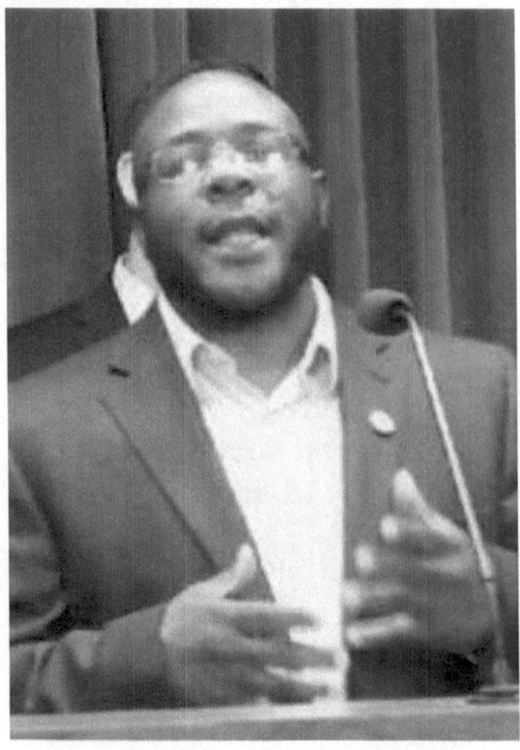

In Memory of my Beloved Canine Son
Chocolate Pierre Abram
July 14, 2004 --- June 26, 2020

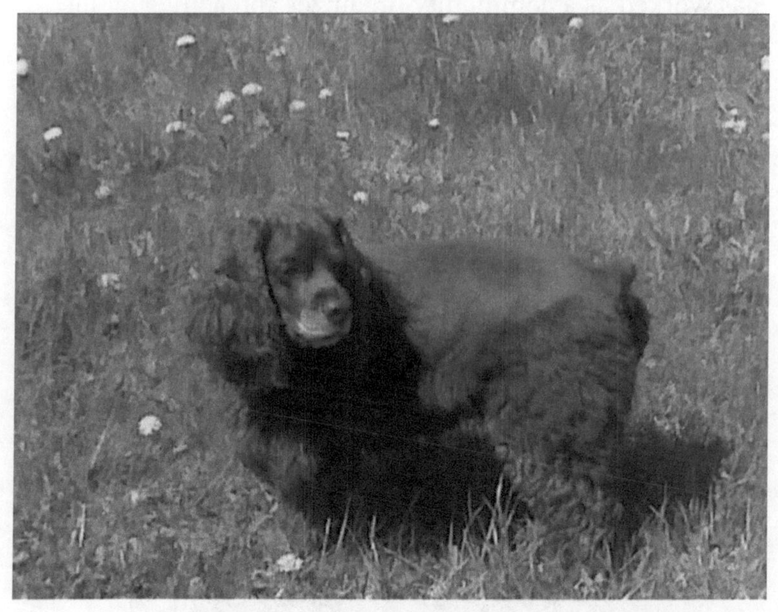

Son, you and I were inseparable for sixteen years.

*Thank you for your unconditional
love, lessons, and legacy. You were my therapy.*

You will FOREVER be a part of me.
I love and miss you so…
Mommy

Mental Health Resources

Dial 911 when in immediate danger

American Foundation for Suicide Prevention
www.afsp.org

American Psychological Association
www.apa.org

Behavior Healthlink
www.behavioralhealthlink.com

Center for Disease Control
www.cdc.gov

Georgia Department of Behavioral Health and
Developmental Disabilities (DBHDD)
https://dbhdd.georgia.gov/

National Alliance on Mental Illness
www.nami.org

Mental Health America
www.mentalhealthamerica.net

National Council for Behavioral Health
https://www.thenationalcouncil.org/

Self-Discovery: Pain, Positioning & Purpose, Inc.
www.sd-ppp.org

Suicide Prevention Lifeline
www.suicidepreventionlifeline.org

Substance Abuse and Mental Health Services Administration
www.samhsa.gov

The Respect Institute
www.dbhdd.georgia.gov

Viewpoint Health
https://www.myviewpointhealth.org/

United Suicide Survivors International
https://unitesurvivors.org/about/

World Health Organization
https://www.who.int/mental_health/prevention/suicide/suicideprevent/en/

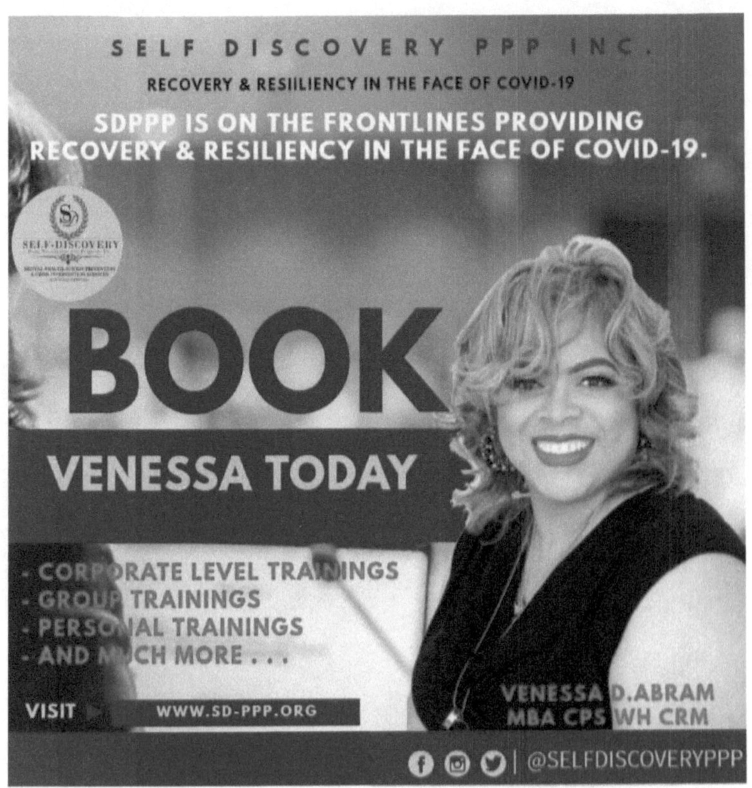

For Bookings, please visit
www.sdp3.org

Self-Discovery is a Daily Journey!

There is <u>No HEALTH</u> without <u>MENTAL HEALTH</u>!

No Shame. No Silence.

No Stigma. No Suicide.

www.ingramcontent.com/pod-product-compliance
Lightning Source LLC
Chambersburg PA
CBHW051452250726
48655CB00001B/367